C O L O U R

HIV Infection and AIDS

Martin A. Birchall MA(Hons) FRCS FRCS (Otol)

Research Fellow in Respiratory Medicine
Royal Postgraduate Medical School, London
Senior Registrar in ENT Surgery
Hammersmith Hospital, London
Registrar in ENT Surgery
St Mary's Hospital, London

Siobhan M. Murphy MRCP

Consultant in Genitourinary Medicine
St Mary's Hospital, London
Consultant in Genitourinary Medicine
Central Middlesex Hospital, London

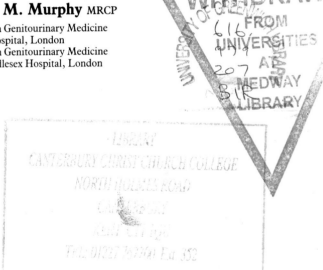

Churchill Livingstone

EDINBURGH LONDON MADRID MELBOURNE NEW YORK AND TOKYO 1992

CHURCHILL LIVINGSTONE
Medical Division of Longman Group Limited

Distributed in the United States of America by
Churchill Livingstone Inc., 650 Avenue of the Americas,
New York, N.Y. 10011, and by associated companies,
branches and representatives throughout the world.

© Longman Group Limited 1992

© Illustrations
St Mary's Hospital Medical School: Figures 6,8,11,12,13,14,15,
16,17,19,22,23,24,26,28,30,31,33,34,35,40,43,49,57,63,65,70,
71,72,73,75,76,77,79,80,102,107,112,116,117,142.
Western Ophthalmic Hospital: Figures 120,121,122,123.

First published 1992
  Reprinted 1995

ISBN 0-443-04578-X

British Library Cataloguing in Publication Data
A catalogue record for this book is available from the British
Library.

Library of Congress Cataloging in Publication Data
A catalogue record for this book is available from the Library of
Congress

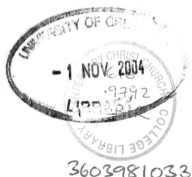

Publisher
Michael Parkinson
Project Editor
Jim Killgore
Production
Nancy Henry
Designer
Design Resources Unit
Sales Promotion Executiv
Marion Pollock

The
publisher's
policy is to use
paper manufactured
from sustainable forests

Printed in Hong Kong
LYP/02

Preface

The clinical problem of HIV infection represents one of the biggest challenges now facing health service workers everywhere. In one decade, it has spread to become a major cause of premature death in some parts of the world. The terms 'HIV infection' and 'AIDS' now appear on most lists of differential diagnoses, making it essential for all health workers to become familiar with its clinical manifestations.

This book is intended to give an overview of the clinical features of HIV infection and AIDS. In the interests of clarity, it has become necessary to omit much information, for which readers are referred to more detailed texts on the subject. It must be emphasized that much of our understanding of HIV infection, particularly those aspects relating to epidemiology, treatment and progression in children, are the subject of continuing research and review and so some statements contained herein may become superseded in time.

This book is dedicated to the memory of those patients who contributed to this volume and who were, sadly, unable to see its completion.

London   M.A.B.
1992   S.M.M.

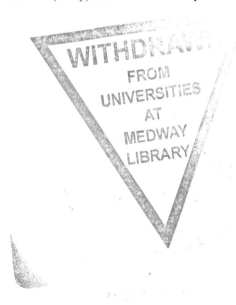

Acknowledgements

We are indebted for much of this book to a series of specialist advisors, all of whom freely provided us with their time, advice and slides from their personal collections:

- African AIDS: Dr Chris Conlon
- Chest medicine: Dr Greg Mason
- Dermatology: Dr Jonathon Leonard
- ENT surgery: Mr Nick Stafford
- Genitourinary medicine: Dr David Tomlinson
- Histopathology: Dr Francesco Scaravelli and Dr Kim Suvarna
- Kaposi's sarcoma: Dr Simon Stewart
- Neurology: Dr John Winer
- Opthalmology: Mr Clive Migdal
- Paediatrics: Dr Sam Walters
- Radiology: Dr Moira McCarthy.

The following also contributed pictures: Dr C. Amerasinghe, Abbott Diagnostics Ltd, Dr G. Bellingham, Blackwell Scientific Pub., Dr P. Dickman, Miss C. Donegan, Dr A. Hines, Dr J.M. Jacobs, Dr R. Lau, Dr R. Logan, Dr F. Moss, Dr B. Peters, Mr M. Savage, Dr J. Selles, Mr D. Simmonds, Dr S. Soucek, Mr A. Tanner, Westway Graphics and Wolfe Publishing Ltd. We are indebted to the Medical Illustration Department of St. Mary's Hospital Medical School for permission to use slides from their collection, and for their expert assistance throughout in the preparation of this book.

London   M.A.B.
1992   S.M.M.

Contents

1 / **Appearance of AIDS**

Early recognition
By the end of 1990, there had been over 300 000 cases of the acquired immunodeficiency syndrome (AIDS) reported to the World Health Organisation (WHO), of which about 4000 were in the UK. The first reported cases of AIDS were in June 1981, when five cases of *Pneumocystis carinii* pneumonia (PCP) in homosexual Californian men were described. One month later, 26 cases of unusually aggressive Kaposi's sarcoma in homosexual men, some of whom also had PCP, were reported in New York. By the end of 1982, it was clear that an outbreak of a new acquired immunodeficiency syndrome had occurred. It appeared to involve a transmissible agent, and the disease was not only confined to homosexual men and intravenous drug abusers.

Origins of the AIDS epidemic
In retrospect, cases of AIDS were seen first in Africa in the 1970s. It is probable that the virus originated there and was transmitted to the United States via Haiti and other island resorts frequented by the US homosexual community. It may have originated by mutation of a related simian immunodeficiency virus prevalent in central Africa.

Distribution of HIV infection
The highest rates of infection are seen in Central African and Caribbean countries (Fig. 1). However, under-reporting is extensive, especially in Africa, and there are an estimated 10 to 20 cases of HIV seropositivity for every case of frank AIDS.

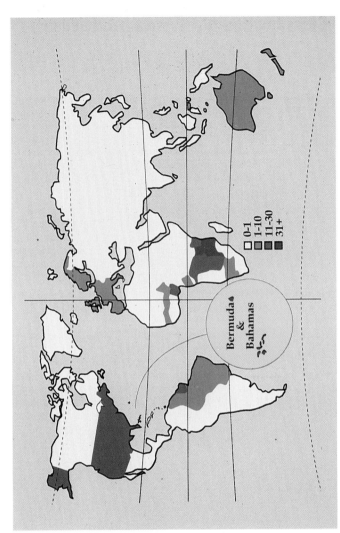

0-1
1-10
11-30
31+

Bermuda
&
Bahamas

Fig. 1 Cumulative AIDS cases reported to the WHO as of March 1991: rates per 100 000 population

2 / Classification of HIV-related disease

Early classification

AIDS and ARC

The Centers for Disease Control in America originally defined AIDS as occurring in a person with a reliably diagnosed disease that is at least moderately indicative of an underlying cellular immune deficiency, and who has no known underlying cause of cellular immune deficiency. AIDS-related complex (ARC) comprised oral candidiasis and constitutional symptoms.

Current classification

CDC Groups

With the development of accurate laboratory tests and increased awareness of the clinical spectrum, modifications of classification became necessary (Fig. 2). In children, certain specific lung conditions (recurrent bacterial infections, lymphocytic interstitial pneumonitis) are also indicator diseases for AIDS (see p. 105).

Pathogenesis of immuno-deficiency

HIV belongs to a group of RNA viruses (retroviruses) which possess an enzyme, reverse transcriptase. This allows DNA to be produced from virus RNA. HIV enters cells by attaching itself to the CD4 antigen present mainly on T4 (helper or inducer) lymphocytes (Fig. 3). Once inside the cell, the virus replicates. Continuous viral replication over time diminishes the pool of T4 cells with consequent disturbance of cell-mediated immunity (Fig. 3). Possibly 60% of HIV-infected individuals will develop AIDS, after a variable latency period averaging about 8 years.

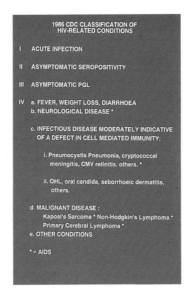

Fig. 2 Centers for Disease Control (CDC) classification of HIV-related disease (1986).

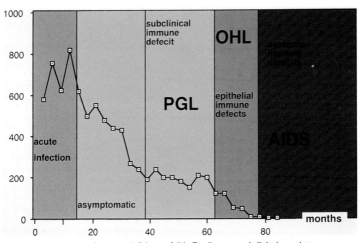

Fig. 3 Progress of immunodeficiency: fall in T-cell count and clinical correlates.

3 / **Routes of infection**

Risk groups Early evidence delineated certain groups particularly
at risk: homosexual men, intravenous drug-users,
haemophiliacs and people of Haitian origin. A more
complete list of groups at risk may now be assembled,
based on improved knowledge of the spread of HIV-
related disease (Fig. 4).

Identification of individuals at risk is sometimes simple
on the basis of history or examination (Fig. 5, & Fig. 6,
p. 8), but some seropositive individuals may not fall
obviously into any of the recognized groups.

Distribution HIV has been isolated from most body fluids including
blood, semen, cervical secretions, breast milk,
cerebrospinal fluid, saliva and tears. Of these, blood,
semen and cervical secretions are particularly infectious,
whilst maternal transmission via milk may represent a
further significant source worldwide. Saliva, in fact,
contains substances inhibitory to HIV replication, and
so transmission by this route seems less likely. The
importance of transmission via heterosexual contact is
increasingly emphasized.

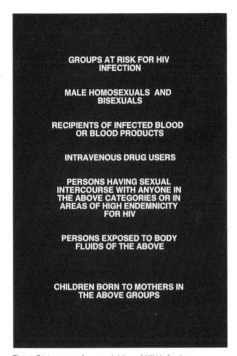

Fig. 4 Risk groups for acquisition of HIV infection.

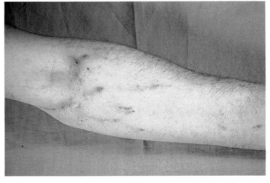

Fig. 5 Puncture marks in a young intravenous drug-user.

4 / **Diagnosis of HIV infection**

When there is clinical suspicion of HIV infection, confirmatory tests are required. It is standard practice in the UK to undertake HIV pre-test counselling whereby the medical, social, employment and insurance implications of a positive HIV antibody test are explained. This is performed by trained medical staff or counsellors. Equally important is the involvement of the counsellor in the psychological support required after a positive diagnosis.

Clinical diagnosis

This is based on the diagnosis of one of the indicator diseases described elsewhere. Three groups of patients are recognized:

- those with an indicator disease but not laboratory tested
- those with positive testing, regardless of clinical picture
- those with laboratory evidence against infection, but unequivocal AIDS clinically.

Laboratory tests

Tests for antibody. Antibody appears 3 weeks to 3 months after exposure and may be reliably detected after this time by a variety of commercial kits. Employing antigen derived from genetic engineering, these mainly utilize enzyme-linked immunosorbant assay (ELISA), and a positive result causes a colour change (Fig. 7). Most centres now use a combined test for detection of both HIV I and II, and positive results may be confirmed by Western blot.

Tests for antigen. These tests mainly look for the core antigen p24 and are useful in the period before antibody becomes detectable.

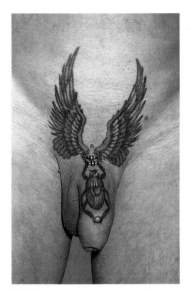

Fig. 6 There are sometimes overt signs of high-risk behaviour, such as this tattoo.

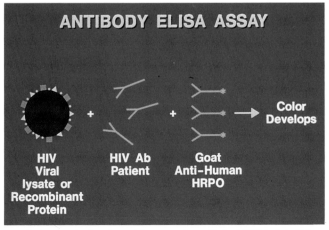

Fig. 7 Mechanism of action of one of the commonly used indirect ELISA tests for HIV antibody.

5 / **Early clinical features**

Acute infection (CDC group I)

Incidence In most cases, seroconversion probably passes unnoticed.

Clinical features Symptomatic seroconversion may present as:

- *Glandular-fever-like illness* comprising sore throat, fever, malaise, lethargy and lymphadenopathy (Fig. 8).
- *Acute, reversible encephalopathy*. This comprises disorientation, loss of memory and altered personality and conscious level.
- *Acute meningoencephalitis* may occur with features of meningeal irritation and drowsiness.
- *Acute myelopathy and neuropathy* has also been reported.

Asymptomatic infection (CDC group II)

Clinical features Not all those who seroconvert enter a phase of chronic infection, but even those with latent infection are probably infectious. Group II disease may last from 2 to 20 years.

Constitutional disease (CDC group IVa)

Clinical features The onset of late disease is often heralded by non-specific clinical features:

- fever for more than one month
- involuntary weight loss of at least 10% of baseline (Fig. 9)
- diarrhoea for more than one month in the absence of any other proven cause.

These symptoms tend to be recurrent features as immunodeficiency advances.

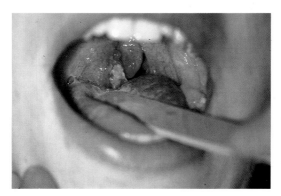

Fig. 8 Acute seroconversion presenting as a glandular-fever-like tonsillitis.

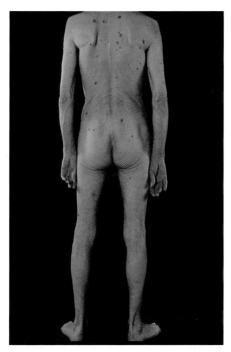

Fig. 9 Cachexia in HIV infection.

Persistent generalized lymphadenopathy (PGL; CDC group III)

Definition A patient having unexplained lymphadenopathy of 3 or more months duration, involving two or more extra-inguinal sites is said to have PGL.

Pathology Histologically, there is mixed follicular hyperplasia and involution, followed by lymphocyte depletion as disease progresses (Fig. 10).

Clinical features There is axillary involvement in 98% of cases, and 86% of these involve cervical chains where enlargement is frequently symmetrical (Fig. 11). Splenic and adenoidal enlargement are variably associated. The nodes are usually greater than 1 cm in diameter and may fluctuate in size. PGL is often present for 6 months or more before medical help is sought. There may be constitutional disturbance as above, and, occasionally, PGL is associated with a Sjögren's-like xerostomia and xerophthalmia.

Differential diagnosis This includes lymphoma, Kaposi's sarcoma and opportunistic infections, such as mycobacteria and any other cause of generalized lymphadenopathy.

Management In most cases, PGL is asymptomatic and requires no treatment. However, where there is any doubt about the diagnosis, especially markedly asymmetrical lymphadenopathy or constitutional disturbance, further investigation is warranted, including fine-needle aspiration and biopsy.

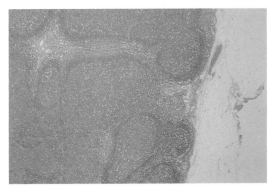

Fig. 10 Lymph node biopsy in PGL: 'geographic' follicular hyperplasia.

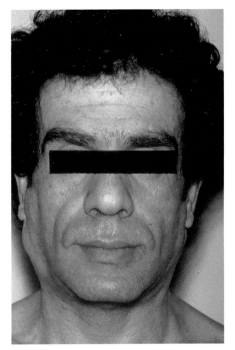

Fig. 11 Bilateral, symmetrical and massive cervical lymphadenopathy in a man with PGL.

Oral candidiasis

The presence of oral candidiasis may be the earliest
clinical sign of immunosuppression that implies HIV
infection in a person with a high risk factor for HIV
infection.

Prevalence Recognized in patients with AIDS since the early 1980s,
oral candidiasis affects between 30% and 90% of HIV-
positive patients.

Clinical features The commonest appearance is the pseudomembranous
form: a creamy plaque that may be wiped off to leave a
bleeding surface (Fig. 12). Erythematous, or atrophic,
candidiasis appears as red patches (Fig. 13), whilst
leukoplakic candidiasis is white and firm and cannot be
wiped off (Fig. 14). Angular cheilitis is a common
perioral manifestation.

Differential diagnosis Candidiasis requires to be differentiated from the various
forms of leukoplakia, especially oral hairy leukoplakia
(OHL; see p. 19). Unlike leukoplakia, scraping with
a tongue depressor will remove candida in most cases.
Where scrapings are possible, the finding of hyphae on
microscopy will confirm a diagnosis of candida. In an
older patient, leukoplakia may represent dysplasia and
a biopsy would be indicated.

Management Treatment may be with topical agents (e.g. nystatin
mouthwashes, amphotericin lozenges). If there is
associated oesophageal candida, systemic antifungals
(e.g. ketoconazole) are required.

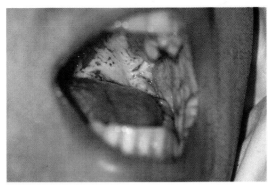

Fig. 12 Gross pseudomembranous candidiasis of oral cavity.

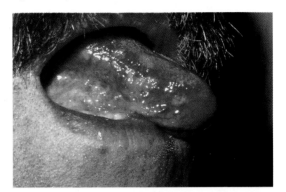

Fig. 13 Painful, red tongue in atrophic candidiasis.

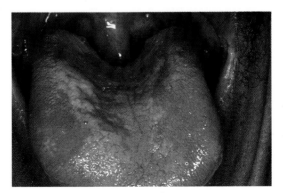

Fig. 14 Mixed leukoplakic and atrophic candidiasis in a patient with AIDS.

Seborrhoeic dermatitis

This affects all groups of HIV-positive patients, and may be a presenting feature. About 80% of patients with AIDS are subject to the condition at some time.

Aetiology

This is unknown. Genetic predisposition is probably relevant, and infection with *Pityrosporum* species has been implicated.

Clinical features

Seborrhoeic dermatitis consists of a red, scaly rash most frequently affecting the cheeks, nasolabial folds, eyebrows and eyelids (Fig. 15). Thus, cosmetic disability can be great. The trunk and intertriginous areas may be involved.

Management

Treatment is with topical steroid preparations, such as hydrocortisone, and antifungals, such as miconazole nitrate. Combination preparations of hydrocortisone and imidazole are useful. In resistant cases, systemic tetracycline may be added. In any case, treatment is only suppressive and needs to be continued indefinitely.

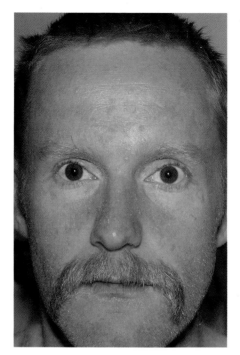

Fig. 15 Scaly rash of facial seborrhoeic dermatitis in a man with PCP.

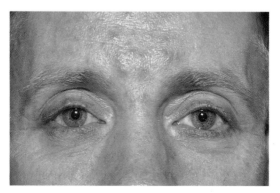

Fig. 16 Follicular blepharitis and acneiform folliculitis of forehead.

Folliculitis

Aetiology In acute folliculitis, *Staphylococcus aureus* may be cultured. Biopsies of chronic lesions may show *Pityrosporum* yeasts within hair follicles. The cause of acneiform folliculitis is unclear, and culture of these lesions results in no growth.

Clinical features Lesions consist of multiple slightly raised papules closely associated with hair follicles. They may occur on any hair-bearing site, though the upper trunk, neck (Fig. 17), limbs (Fig. 18) and intertriginous areas are most commonly affected. Acneiform folliculitis is characterized by a variety of particularly pruritic follicular lesions varying in distribution and degree (Fig. 16, p. 16, and Fig. 19).

Management Long-term, systemic antibiotics and antifungals may be tried, but the condition is usually refractory.

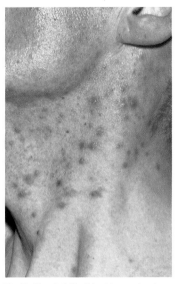

Fig. 17 Chronic folliculitis of face and neck.

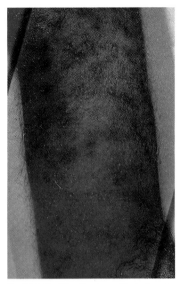

Fig. 18 Folliculitis of leg in a patient who was also a nasal carrier of *Staphylococcus aureus*.

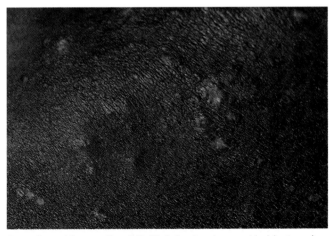

Fig. 19 Some of these acneiform folliculitis lesions have been scratched due to pruritus.

6 / **Oral hairy leukoplakia**

Oral hairy leukoplakia (OHL) has been regarded for some time now as pathognomonic for AIDS. Although occasionally seen in immunosuppressed transplant recipients, it is only since the advent of HIV that the condition has been characterized.

Incidence It affects about 20% of HIV patients and is a presenting feature in 5%, making its recognition of great importance to all medical and dental personnel.

Pathology Originally thought to be due to the human papilloma virus, it is now known to represent an opportunistic infection by the Epstein–Barr virus (EBV) within the mucosa of the oral cavity. Histologically, OHL is characterized by epithelial hyperparakeratosis with balloon cells and keratin hairs. There is a lack of inflammatory response in 86% (Fig. 20). By special staining, the virus can be visualized in various stages of replication within the epithelium (Fig. 21). The characteristic location of OHL may be due to secretion of EBV by the salivary glands.

Prognosis Although a benign condition, OHL has a very high positive predictive value for the presence of HIV infection, and 83% of subjects develop AIDS within 3 years.

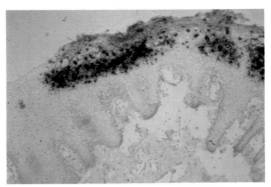

Fig. 20 Section of OHL showing hyperparakeratosis and balloon cells. In-situ hybridization shows EBV.

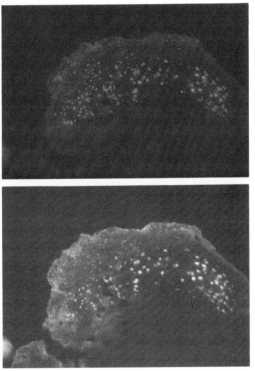

Fig. 21 Radioimmunofluorescent images: early antigen (green) and viral capsid antigen (red).

Clinical features **Symptoms.** OHL is usually asymptomatic. Any discomfort is often due to the presence of an intercurrent candidal or other infection. It may spontaneously regress and relapse.

Signs. Early OHL appears as isolated, often unilateral whitish patches on the sides of the tongue (Fig. 22). Later, it may become raised, corrugated, shaggy or remain flat. The commonest site is the lateral border of the tongue, but the dorsum of the tongue (Fig. 23), the floor of the mouth (Fig. 24), the cheeks and palate are all variably affected. In the most severe cases, OHL may take on a yellow or brownish appearance due to the drying of keratin (Fig. 23).

Differential diagnosis OHL needs to be differentiated from oral candida with which it is often associated (see p. 13). Leukoplakia in sites atypical for OHL may represent dysplasia or neoplasia and thus warrant biopsy.

Management The majority of cases require no specific treatment. If discomfort is present, it should be treated as oral candidiasis initially. The occasional patient may request treatment on cosmetic grounds. Oral acyclovir can be used, although recurrence is the rule. OHL may regress with zidovudine treatment.

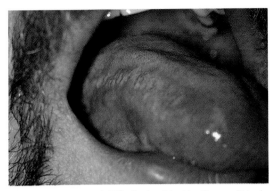

Fig. 22 A patient with early OHL affecting right side of tongue. Note also aphthous ulcers.

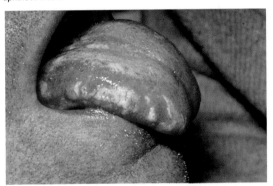

Fig. 23 Extensive OHL on sides and dorsum of tongue.

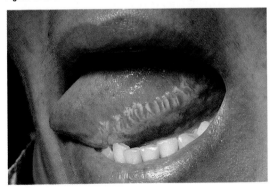

Fig. 24 A patient with AIDS: typical corrugations blend with flat OHL on the floor of the mouth.

7 / Infective skin lesions

In the initial management of any patient with HIV infection, the skin and mucous membranes represent easily accessible areas to examine and biopsy. They may present with common skin infections which are more extensive or recurrent than usual, or with opportunistic infectious lesions from which a diagnosis of AIDS or AIDS-related disease can be made.

Wart virus

Clinical features Wart virus infection, including the sexually acquired form, is very common in HIV infection. Verrucous lesions may be unusally extensive, or occur in unusual sites (Fig. 57, p. 48). There is rarely any doubt about the diagnosis (Fig. 25).

Management Topical treatment with keratolytics or cryotherapy is useful for cosmetically disabling lesions.

Herpes zoster

Clinical features This is often multidermatomal (Fig. 26) and protracted. On healing, post-herpetic neuralgia or cosmetically damaging scarring may occur (Fig. 27).

Management Given early, high-dose intravenous or oral acyclovir may limit spread. Adequate analgesia is essential. Maintenance acyclovir may be required.

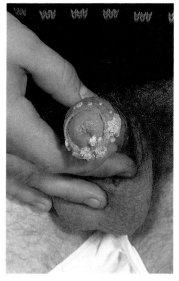

Fig. 25 Multiple warts of the penis.

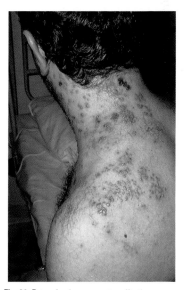

Fig. 26 Extensive herpes zoster affecting dermatomes C2 to C4.

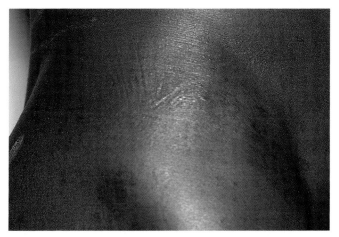

Fig. 27 Hypertrophic scarring and depigmentation following herpes zoster in AIDS.

Herpes simplex

Clinical features In addition to the features described on page 77, herpes simplex may give rise to giant or chronic skin lesions (Fig. 28).

Management Where diagnosis has been confirmed by viral culture or biopsy, acyclovir therapy is effective against chronic lesions.

Molluscum contagiosum

Aetiology This represents infection with a pox virus, and occurs in up to 18% of patients with AIDS. It is spread by close physical contact.

Clinical features Lesions are painless, pearly and umbilicated papules which may be very extensive (Fig. 29).

Management If treatment is required for cosmetic purposes, cryotherapy or topical phenol may effect cure, but recurrence is common.

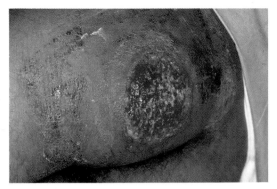

Fig. 28 Giant herpetic ulcer, from which HSV I was cultured. The lesion responded to acyclovir.

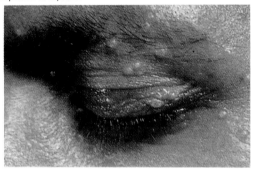

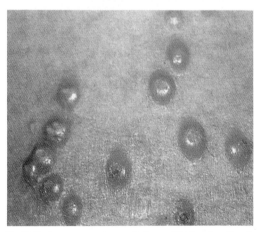

Fig. 29 Molluscum contagiosum affecting eyelid (above) and face (b elow).

Candidiasis

Intertrigo and mucocutaneous candidiasis are described elsewhere (see p. 13).

Dermatophytoses

Clinical features These infections are all common and spread rapidly. Tinea pedis affects the feet, and *trichophytum rubrum* affects the trunk and limbs. Onychomycosis, usually due to candidiasis, is common (Fig. 30).

Diagnosis Hyphae may be demonstrated on potassium hydroxide preparation of scrapings or biopsies. Fungal culture may be necessary to select the best treatment.

Management Topical therapy, e.g. with clotrimazole cream, should be tried, but unusually extensive or recurrent infections may require systemic ketoconazole.

Other opportunistic skin infections

Clinical features As part of disseminated opportunistic systemic infections, e.g. pneumocystosis, candidiasis, cryptococcosis or histoplasmosis (Figs 31 & 32), skin lesions may occur. Where doubt exists, biopsy should be performed.

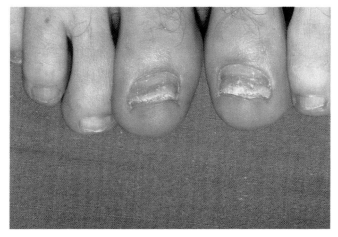

Fig. 30 Onychomycosis of feet.

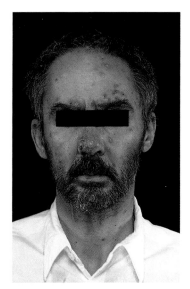

Fig. 31 Crusted facial papules in disseminated histoplasmosis.

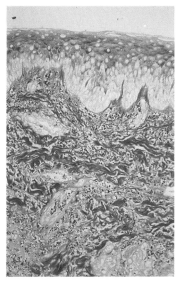

Fig. 32 Biopsy of lesion in Figure 31 with black-staining fungal spores.

Bacterial infection

Clinical features   In addition to staphylococcal infection (see p. 17), skin lesions may be associated with septicaemia, such as salmonellosis. Staphylococcal lesions may be unusually recurrent (Fig. 33).

Mycobacteria

Clinical features   Tuberculous lymphadenitis (Fig. 49, p. 42, and Fig. 134, p. 110) may involve the skin (e.g. 'collar-stud abscess'). In addition, there may be direct involvement producing violaceous lesions of lupus vulgaris (Fig. 34). *Mycobacterium avium-intracellulare* (MAI), *M. kansasii* and *M. haemophilum* are sometimes also seen in this context.

Management   As with mycobacterial infection elsewhere, triple therapy should be instituted.

Non-infective skin conditions

Seborrhoeic dermatitis is described above (p. 15).

Vasculitis
Disseminated purpuric rashes are common. The aetiology is unknown.

Drug reactions

Clinical features   HIV-infected individuals are particularly liable to allergic reactions, which may take any form from red maculopapular eruptions (Fig. 35) to severe Stevens–Johnson-type reactions.

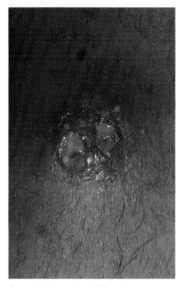

Fig. 33 Ecthyma in an AIDS patient.

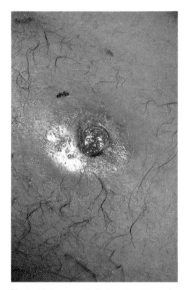

Fig. 34 Violaceous skin lesion, the culture of which produced mycobacteria.

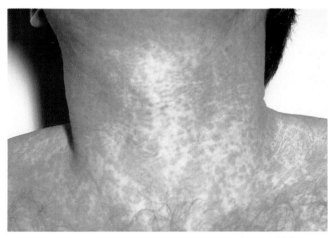

Fig. 35 Erythematous maculopapular reaction to septrin in a patient with AIDS.

8 / Kaposi's sarcoma (KS)

Until the advent of AIDS, the tumour first described by Moritz Kaposi in 1872 remained rare. However, it is now one of the commonest index conditions of AIDS and its recognition has attained considerable importance.

Incidence   This varies depending on the risk group considered:
- *homosexual men* 21%
- *transfusion and drug-related* 3–4%
- *haemophiliacs* less than 1%.

The incidence in homosexual AIDS cases appears to be declining.

Aetiology   KS is associated with cellular immunodeficiency. Certain HIV proteins have the ability to promote growth in KS cells in vitro, but there is some evidence of an associated transmissible agent other than HIV. In addition, genetic predisposition (e.g. HLA-DR3) and male gender play a part.

Pathology   Histologically, KS consists of collections of endothelial-lined spaces separated by proliferating spindle cells (Fig. 36). The condition is invariably multifocal (Fig. 37).

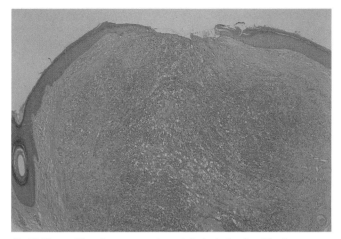

Fig. 36 Ulcerated Kaposi's sarcoma and vascularized spindle cell proliferation.

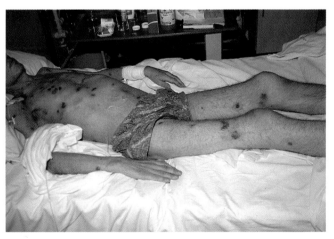

Fig. 37 Disseminated KS of trunk and limbs.

Clinical features　KS may occur in the later stages of HIV infection, and therefore is often concurrent with opportunistic infections and other features of AIDS. Early lesions (patch stage) are quite innocous in appearance and somewhat resemble bruises (Fig. 38). Plaque stage lesions are less diffuse and slightly raised (Fig. 39). Later, lesions become nodular (Fig. 40) and may ulcerate. In colour, KS varies from pale pink, through violet, to dark brown. Initially, the lower limb is favoured, but KS may occur on any cutaneous surface including mucous membranes (see p. 57). In general, lesions are painless and non-tender, but considerable cosmetic disability often results.

Prognosis　Although normally indolent, when KS disseminates to viscera (see p. 45), serious and life-threatening complications may result. Conversely, lesions may occasionally regress spontaneously.

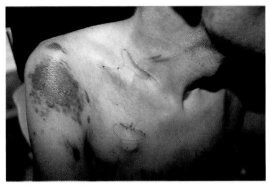

Fig. 38 Patch-stage lesion, showing bruise-like appearance.

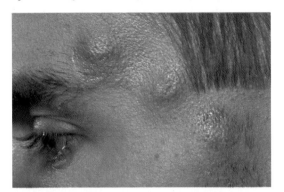

Fig. 39 Multiple, violaceous facial lesions of plaque stage KS.

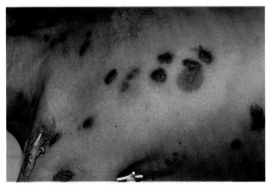

Fig. 40 Dark brown, nodular-stage lesions in advanced AIDS. Some are ulcerated.

Diagnosis In a patient with known AIDS and classical skin lesions, biopsy is generally unnecessary. However, in view of the sometimes innocuous appearances of KS, all dermatological conditions in high-risk individuals need careful scrutiny and consideration for biopsy where doubt remains.

Management Treatment should be reserved for lesions presenting cosmetic disability or complications such as ulceration or bowel or bronchial obstruction. A single treatment of radiotherapy may provide a perfect cosmetic result for early lesions, but late lesions leave haemosiderin 'tattoos' (Fig. 41) after treatment, due to vascular leakage. Radiotherapy is often outstripped by the disease. Systemic therapy with bleomycin and vincristine can be reasonably effective. Alpha-interferon may have an effect in selected patients, but may be associated with not inconsiderable toxicity. The response rate to these agents is short-lived. Indeed, any treatment should be regarded as palliative.

Complications Lesions may ulcerate, and this may be severe (Fig. 42). KS may obstruct viscera, as described above. Lymphatic involvement is common, and lymphoedema may ensue (Fig. 43).

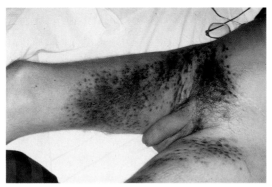

Fig. 41 Hyperpigmentation remaining after radiotherapy for KS of groin.

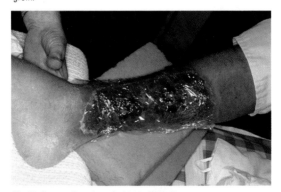

Fig. 42 Severe ulceration of advanced KS of lower limb.

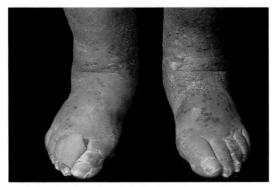

Fig. 43 Lymphoedema of legs following KS involvement of inguinal lymph nodes.

9 / Respiratory manifestations

The lung is the organ most frequently affected in patients with AIDS. The use of prophylaxis against *Pneumocystis carinii* pneumonia is gradually altering the clinical picture.

Pneumocystis carinii pneumonia (PCP)

Pathology

PCP is the commonest index disease for AIDS: 60% of AIDS patients develop PCP at some time. Despite recent debate over taxonomy, *Pneumocystis* is probably best regarded as a fungus. Pneumonia appears to result from reactivation of infection that would be subclinical in the immunocompetent. Attacks may recur, and extrapulmonary disease, though rare, has been described.

Clinical features

Initial symptoms are non-specific: anorexia and fatigue. These characteristically give way to a non-productive cough, low-grade fever and dyspnoea, which eventually occurs at rest. Symptom severity may be affected by the presence of PCP prophylaxis. Even with extensive disease, often the only chest signs are tachycardia and tachypnoea with normal breath sounds. Other signs of HIV infection, such as OHL, may be present.

Investigations

Chest X-Ray. Typical features are shown in Figure 44. Atypical features (Fig. 45) are not unusual, especially with prior PCP prophylaxis. These include: focal lung infiltrates, focal alveolar consolidation, focal nodules with cavitation, and pneumothorax.

Arterial blood gases typically reveal hypoxaemia, but this may only be on exercise in mild cases.

Pulmonary function tests typically show diminished single breath diffusing capacity for carbon monoxide (DLCO) and mild to moderate restriction.

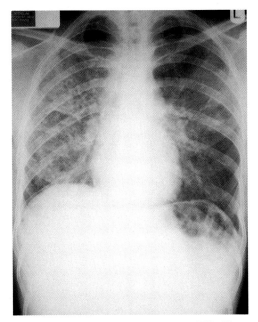

Fig. 44 Typical CXR of a moderately severe case of PCP: diffuse bilateral perihilar infiltrates.

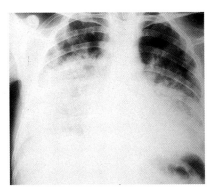

Fig. 45 Advanced PCP with widespread consolidation of mid and lower zones and some apical sparing.

Diagnosis   Many centres will commence therapy for PCP based on the clinical picture outlined above, and will only proceed to further investigations if there is an unsatisfactory response. Sputum induced by the inhalation of 3% nebulized saline can be examined cytologically for pneumocysts. Bronchoscopy and broncho-alveolar lavage (BAL) (Figs 46 & 48), with or without transbronchial biopsy (Fig. 47), may reliably detect pneumocystis.

Treatment   First line therapy for PCP is trimethoprim (50 mg/kg/d) plus sulphamethoxazole (250 mg/kg/d) (co-trimoxazole), intravenously or orally for 21 days. Allergies to this drug are common (Fig. 35), and replacing with the equally effective sulphamethoxazole dapsone (100 mg/d) may be necessary. Aerosolized pentamidine given once daily has been used to treat mild to moderate disease, when the patient is able to effectively receive therapy. Intravenous or intramuscular pentamidine has also been used.

Prophylaxis   The CDC (p. 3) recommend prophylaxis for PCP in any HIV-positive patient whose CD4 lymphocyte count is less than 200 or 20% of total lymphocytes, or after the first attack of PCP. Several prophylactic regimens have been shown to be effective, including low-dose co-trimoxazole 5–7 times a week, nebulized pentamidine 300 mg 2–4 times a month, dapsone 100 mg and pyrimethamine 25 mg once or twice weekly. The choice depends on local resources, and the compliance and allergic profile of the individual patient.

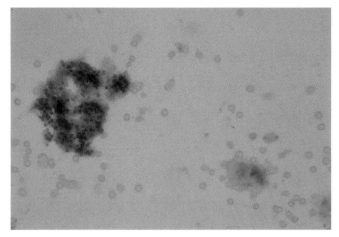

Fig. 46 Grocott's stain of a BAL specimen with pneumocysts staining blue-green.

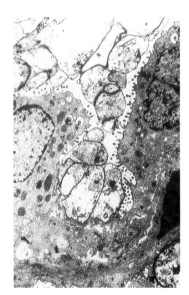

Fig. 47 Electron micrograph in PCP: alveoli full of trophozoites and cyst form inferiorly.

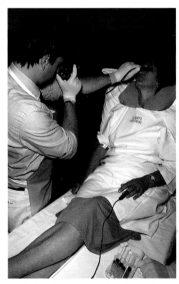

Fig. 48 Bronchoscopy in HIV-positive patient.

Mycobacterium tuberculosis (MTB)

Incidence   MTB affects 2–10% of US AIDS patients and 2–14% of
all patients with HIV in parts of sub-Saharan Africa.
Although only extrapulmonary TB is classified as an
AIDS index disease, it is, in fact, confined to the lungs in
30–50% of cases.

Clinical features   Reactivation of infection is usual, and the clinical picture
depends on the level of immunocompetence. In AIDS,
the course tends to be more typical of progressive primary
disease. Common presenting features are cough, fever,
lymphadenitis (Fig. 49) and weight loss.

Diagnosis   **Common radiographic findings** are hilar or mediastinal
adenopathy and lower or mid-lung field infiltrates. By
contrast with non-HIV patients, apical infiltrates (Fig. 50)
and cavitation are rare. Importantly, CXR may be
entirely normal.

Examination of sputum and BAL (p. 39) for acid-fast
bacilli is useful, and MTB may be subsequently cultured,
even with a normal smear (50% of cases).

Management   This is with 6–9 months of triple therapy: isoniazid
300 mg/d, rifampicin 600 mg/d (450 mg/d if less than 50
kg), pyrazinamide 25 mg/kg/d. Ethambutol 25 mg/kg/d is
used in cases of isoniazid resistance or extrapulmonary
disease. Relapse after conventional therapy is rare.
Regular tuberculin skin-testing may have a role with a
view to prophylactic isoniazid if required, although
allergy is common in HIV infection.

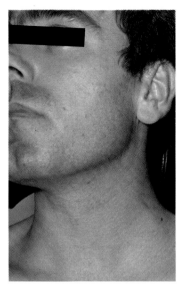

Fig. 49 Extrapulmonary MTB in anterior triangle neck nodes of a Brazilian man with AIDS.

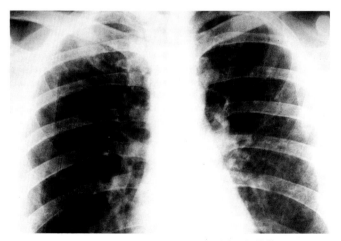

Fig. 50 Chest X-ray in tuberculous lung disease showing right apical infiltrates.

Atypical mycobacteria

MAI, *M.kansasii* and *M.xenopii* are often isolated from the lung in AIDS and may be incidental or part of disseminated disease.

Bacteria

Clinical features   Bacterial pneumonia is more common in patients with AIDS. Patients present with fever, cough, dyspnoea and pleuritic chest pain. After identification of the organism in sputum, the appropriate antibiotic may be instituted. *Haemophilus influenzae* (Fig. 51) is often found.

Cytomegalovirus (CMV)

Pathology   CMV is often a common isolate in PCP, though it is usually thought to represent colonization. CMV may also cause interstitial pneumonia, although this is infrequent in contrast to those immunosuppressed for transplantation.

Clinical features   These include progressive dyspnoea and dry cough, with tachycardia, tachypnoea, hypoxaemia and interstitial infiltrates on CXR.

Fungal infection

Pathology   *Cryptococcus neoformans* can cause pneumonia, often as part of a disseminated infection. Histoplasmosis and coccidiomycosis also occur.

Clinical features   Signs of cryptococcal meningitis (p. 91) may be accompanied by cough, dyspnoea and haemoptysis. CXR shows well-defined nodules which may cavitate, or reticular shadowing (Fig. 52). Treatment is as for central nervous system involvement (p. 91).

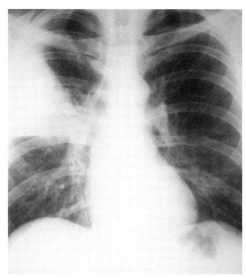

Fig. 51 Right mid-zone consolidation due to *H.influenzae*, which responded to penicillin.

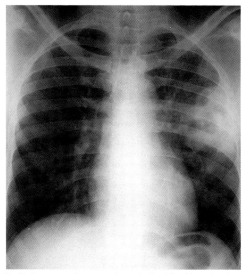

Fig. 52 Cryptococcal pneumonia: cavitating left mid-zone opacity consistent with fungal infection.

Kaposi's sarcoma (KS)

At necropsy, most patients with KS have lung involvement. Better treatment of opportunistic infection has highlighted pulmonary KS as more of a clinical problem.

Clinical features KS may occur anywhere in the respiratory tract, causing obstruction, infection or haemorrhage. Dry cough, dyspnoea, wheeze and haemoptysis are seen. Respiratory failure may ensue.

Diagnosis Nodular shadowing, pleural fluid and hilar adenopathy are seen on CXR (Fig. 53). Bronchoscopic visualization (Fig. 54) suffices for diagnosis if KS is present elsewhere.

Management Radiotherapy or chemotherapy may be used for symptomatic cases.

Lymphoma

Pathology These are almost exclusively non-Hodgkin's B cell in type (Fig. 55). Unlike lymphoma in the general population, intrathoracic involvement is uncommon.

Clinical features Pleural effusions, mediastinal adenopathy and reticulonodular infiltrates occur (Fig. 55).

Lymphocytic interstitial pneumonitis (LIP)

Originally described in children (p. 105), this is now seen in adult AIDS, where some response to steroids has been reported in symptomatic cases.

Cardiac disease

This is rare, but pericarditis is described.

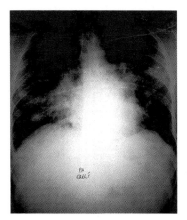

Fig. 53 Lung KS: right basal pleural effusion, coarse consolidation and some bilateral nodules.

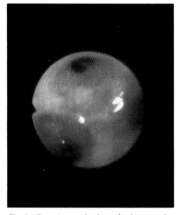

Fig. 54 Bronchoscopic view of submucosal KS in the trachea.

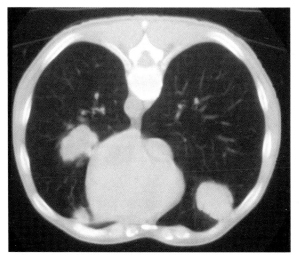

Fig. 55 CT scan in lymphoma with soft tissue lesions in both lung fields.

The external ear suffers from many of the cutaneous conditions common elsewhere in HIV infection. Thus, seborrhoeic dermatitis, molluscum contagiosum, papillomata (Fig. 57) and Kaposi's sarcoma are all common in this site.

Otitis Externa

Aetiology This may be idiopathic or secondary to otitis media, dermatitis or obstruction, e.g. by Kaposi's sarcoma.

Pathology Common infecting organisms are *Pseudomonas aeruginosa* and *proteus*. However, fungal infections such as *Aspergillus* do occur and can be very aggressive. *Pneumocystis carinii* has also been a reported cause.

Clinical features **Symptoms** are pain, discharge and deafness.

Signs. Otoscopy reveals a cream coloured discharge usually obscuring the tympanic membrane (Fig. 56). An underlying cause, such as tumour or dermatitis, may be observed. Bacterial infection may spread causing cellulitis of the adjacent pinna.

Management It is essential to send swabs for bacteriological and fungal microscopy and culture. Treatment should begin with aural toilet, aminoglycoside ear drops and analgesia. If cellulitis intervenes, intravenous benzyl penicillin and flucloxacillin are indicated. Any underlying cause should then be managed appropriately: dermatitis with topical steroids, and Kaposi's sarcoma with the Argon laser.

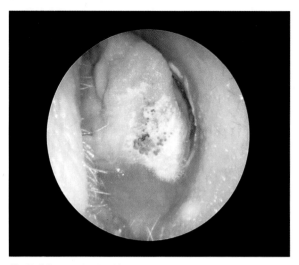

Fig. 56 Yellow exudate in otitis externa with black spores of *Aspergillus niger* visible.

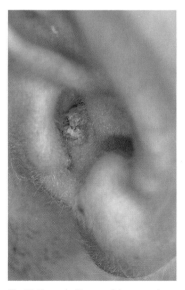

Fig. 57 These papillomata of the external ear were successfully treated by cryotherapy.

11 / **Middle ear**

Otitis media

Aetiology   This may be a primary infection, or there may be a pre-existing condition such as perforation. Eustachian tube dysfunction secondary to benign follicular hypertrophy of the adenoids (Fig. 58), nasopharyngeal tumour, or upper respiratory tract infection has led to an increase in serous otitis media (glue ear; Fig. 59) in HIV infection.

Pathology   The effusion of serous otitis media contains few bacilli, but the HIV has been cultured within it. *S.pneumoniae*, *H. influenzae*, *Pneumocystis* and *Cryptococcus* have been found in acute infections.

Clinical features   **Serous otitis media** presents with conductive deafness, and there may be a mass of adenoidal tissue in the postnasal space.
Acute otitis media presents with acute pain, deafness and unsteadiness. There is a red drum on otoscopy. Otorrhoea may ensue.

Management   Serous otitis requires ephedrine nosedrops 1%, and attention to underlying pathology: adenoidal blockage may be so marked as to require curettage for relief of symptoms and to exclude lymphoma. Failure of the effusion to resolve may require grommet insertion. In acute otitis media, oral amoxycillin and analgesia are prescribed. Failure to resolve in 48 hr necessitates myringotomy and drainage, remembering to send pus for culture.

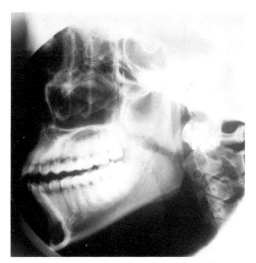

Fig. 58 Adenoidal enlargement shown on lateral neck X-ray.

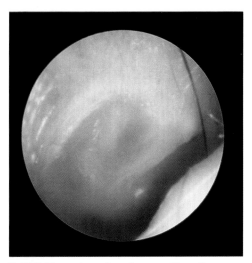

Fig. 59 Dull tympanic membrane in serous otitis media associated with adenoidal enlargement.

12 / Inner ear

Sensorineural deafness

Aetiology

This has many potential causes: infections such as syphilis, cerebral CMV (p. 93), cryptococcosis and toxoplasmosis, ototoxic medications, especially aminoglycosides and cytotoxics, and cerebral tumours. It is possible that primary HIV deafness occurs as part of generalized encephalopathy.

Investigations

This should include syphilis and toxoplasma serology and viral titres. Pure tone audiometry may show high-frequency loss (Fig. 60), and brainstem evoked responses may help to localize a lesion. If there is no obvious cause, an MRI scan is indicated.

Management

The underlying cause should be treated, but despite this, most cases do not improve and an hearing aid may be required.

Herpes zoster oticus

A common site of herpes zoster infection in HIV patients is the inner ear, causing the Ramsay–Hunt syndrome.

Clinical features

There is acute onset of severe pain with vertigo, deafness and a lower motor neurone facial palsy of variable severity. This is followed 24–48 hours later by a rash, often multidermatomal (Fig. 26, p. 24), and otoscopy may reveal vesicles (Fig. 61).

Management

Prostration may require intravenous fluids, vestibular sedatives and strong analgesia. Acyclovir should be commenced as soon as vesicles appear.

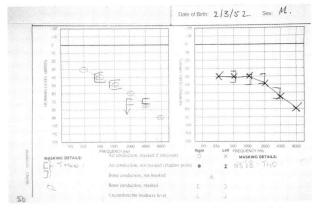

Date of Birth: 2/3/52 Sex: M.

Fig. 60 Pure-tone audiogram showing high-tone sensorineural hearing loss.

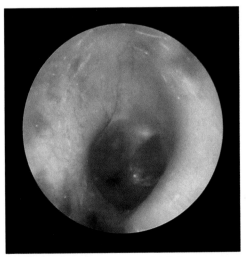

Fig. 61 Segmental vesiculation postero-inferiorly on otoscopy in Ramsay–Hunt syndrome.

13 / Nose and sinuses

Chronic rhinosinusitis

This is very common in HIV infection, and may have an allergic basis. Candidiasis also occurs here.

Clinical features   These include rhinorrhoea, which may be purulent, and nasal obstruction of variable severity.

Managment   Rhinoscopy, preferably with a flexible nasendoscope, is used to exclude obstructive lesions, e.g. Kaposi's sarcoma and lymphoma. Swabs are taken for bacterial and fungal culture. Oral ketoconazole is used to treat candidiasis, otherwise empirical treatment is with steroid sprays.

Acute sinusitis

Pathology   There is most often a mixed aerobic and anaerobic infection. Patients with AIDS may also harbour fungi, mycobacteria and *Legionella*, and the sinuses may act as a reservoir of such infections.

Clinical features   Acute pain and tenderness occurs around the cheek and orbit, with periorbital oedema (Fig. 62). Sinus X-ray may show a fluid level or opacity (Fig. 63).

Management   An antral washout provides symptomatic relief. The aspirate should be sent for culture. A broad-spectrum antibiotic and anti-fungal should be used, preferably intravenously.

External nose

This is a common site for KS (Fig. 64).

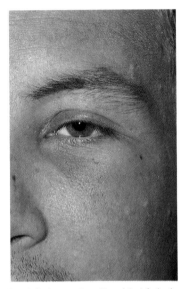

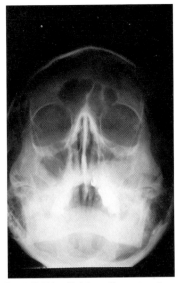

Fig. 62 Redness and swelling of the left cheek in acute sinusitis in an AIDS patient.

Fig. 63 Fluid level in left maxillary antrum is visible on this sinus X-ray of the same patient.

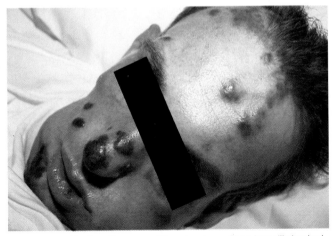

Fig. 64 Gross nodular Kaposi's sarcoma of the external nose. The submandibular gland is also involved.

14 / Oral cavity

The commonest oral manifestations of HIV infection are candidiasis and hairy oral leukoplakia (see pp. 13, 14, and 19–22). However, other manifestations may arise in this site.

Herpes simplex (HSV)

Clinical features Generally, this is self-limiting with restricted areas of vesiculation and ulceration healing in 7–10 days. With immunosuppression, this may become more generalized, especially in perioral (Figs 65 & 66) and palatal (Fig. 67) regions, requiring oral acyclovir.

Other viruses

Clinical features Cytomegalovirus (CMV) may cause ulceration clinically indistinguishable from aphthous ulceration (Fig. 71), whilst the warty condylomata acuminata of human papilloma virus have also been observed. Herpes zoster rarely involves the mouth.

Management Any oral lesion not responding to simple therapy should be considered for biopsy. Culture of virus or demonstration of inclusion bodies are indications for antiviral therapy.

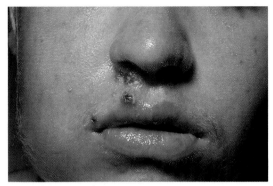

Fig. 65 Multiple perioral vesicles of HSV I.

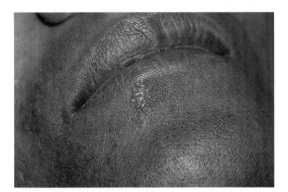

Fig. 66 Perioral vesicles producing HSV II on culture.

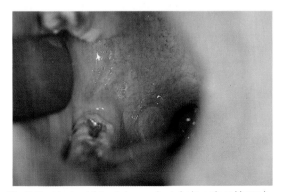

Fig. 67 Persistent, painful oral ulcer proving to be herpetic on biopsy. It responded to acyclovir.

Kaposi's sarcoma

This is a common site for presentation of Kaposi's sarcomata.

Clinical features Early lesions are flat and bruise-like and are commonest on the palate (Fig. 68) and gingiva. However, they may become very large and ulcerated (Fig. 69). Symptoms are unusual, but large lesions may cause problems with deglutition or, rarely, airway obstruction.

Diagnosis In the presence of other features of HIV infection and a characteristic appearance, biopsy is usually unnecessary, although it is sometimes required to rule out lymphoma or squamous cell carcinoma.

Management Local radiotherapy (16–20 Gy in 4 fractions) is effective, but troublesome stomatitis often occurs. Therefore, chemotherapy with vincristine and bleomycin is preferred.

Acute necrotizing ulcerative gingivitis (ANUG)

ANUG, or 'trench-mouth', is a bacterial infection which is now rare in the absence of malnutrition, but a similar condition is also seen in patients with HIV infection.

Clinical features Bleeding, painful gums (Fig. 70) that may progress to ulceration and bony destruction.

Management Topical povidone iodine and oral metronidazole are prescribed. Meticulous oral hygiene is necessary.

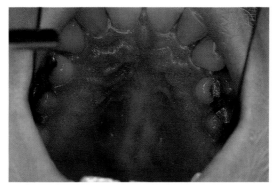

Fig. 68 Bruise-like patch of KS on hard palate.

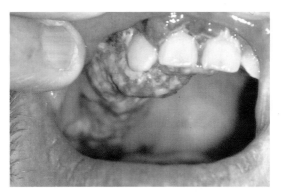

Fig. 69 Necrotic, ulcerating KS of upper jaw.

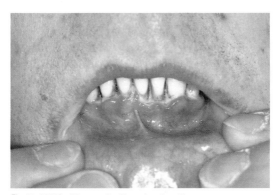

Fig. 70 ANUG with necrosis of interdental papillae

Aphthous ulceration

In HIV infection, these are common and tend to be recurrent and refractory to treatment.

Clinical features Initially small white papules, these break down to form shallow ulcers. They may reach 1 cm or more in size (Fig. 71) and may occasionally become necrotic (Fig. 72), when diagnosis may be difficult. The commonest sites are the lips and buccal mucosa, with tongue and interdental locations being rare. If extensive, aphthous ulcers may interfere with deglutition.

Differential diagnosis Infectious lesions, especially herpes simplex and cytomegalovirus, and neoplastic lesions such as lymphoma or squamous cell carcinoma need to be excluded.

Management Topical steroid preparations (Adcortyl in Orabase) facilitate healing, while lignocaine jelly gives some symptomatic relief. The most severe cases may be helped by the cautious use of thalidomide, taking care to stop if signs of neuropathy occur. Strong analgesia may be necessary for eating. If there is any doubt about the diagnosis, biopsy is mandatory.

Thrombocytopenia

This has been reported in connection with a variety of viral infections, but is particularly common in HIV infection.

Clinical features In the oral cavity, this presents as petechiae, ecchymosis (Fig. 73) or bleeding gums. Treatment is with platelet infusions in severe cases.

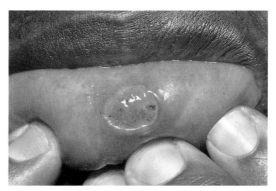

Fig. 71 Large aphthous ulcer of labial mucosa which responded to adcortyl treatment.

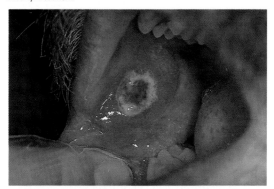

Fig. 72 Necrotic buccal aphthous ulcer.

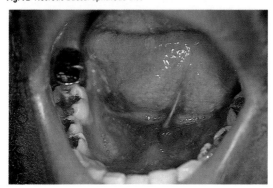

Fig. 73 Sublingual ecchymosis due to thrombocytopenia. Note also angular stomatitis and OHL.

Lymphoma

Pathology As with other AIDS lymphomas, these are non-Hodgkins and poorly differentiated. Some are associated with Epstein–Barr virus infection. Prognosis tends to be poor, although occasional idiosyncratic response to treatment does occur.

Clinical features Lymphoma may present in the tonsil (Figs 74 & 75), alveolus, palate (Fig. 76) or cheek regions. They are painless unless infected but may rapidly ulcerate. It is essential to perform a full physical examination to exclude disseminated disease.

Diagnosis A clinically suspicious lesion should undergo early biopsy, from which the histological features of lymphoma (Fig. 81, p. 66) are sought. A careful programme of investigation including chest X-ray, abdominal CT scan and bone-marrow biopsy is then undertaken to stage the disease.

Management Localized lymphoma can be managed by radiotherapy, but the disease is usually widespread by the time of diagnosis. Hence, chemotherapy, e.g. vincristine and adriamycin, is generally required.

Squamous cell carcinoma

This is the commonest intraoral neoplasm in non-HIV individuals, and may also occur with increased frequency in immunosuppression, including AIDS. The commonest appearance is of an ulcer with raised edges and treatment involves excision or iridium wire implants.

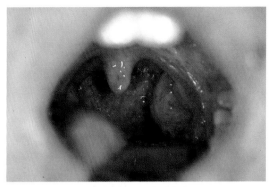

Fig. 74 This non-Hodgkins lymphoma of the left tonsil was the presenting feature of AIDS in this man.

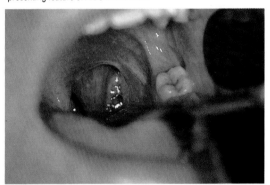

Fig. 75 Local regression followed chemotherapy, but intracranial spread caused death weeks later.

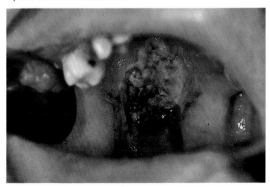

Fig. 76 This lymphoma presented as a necrotic ulcer of the hard palate.

15 / **Salivary glands**

Parotid enlargement

This is a well-recognized presentation of paediatric AIDS (Fig. 130, p. 106), but also occurs in adult disease.

Pathology The commonest condition is cystic enlargement, which may be due to sialadenitis (HIV may be cultured from saliva of infected patients) or may represent cystic degeneration of hyperplastic lymphoid tissue.

Clinical features There is gradual, possibly massive, painless enlargement of the parotid gland (Fig. 77), which may be bilateral.

Differential diagnosis The most important conditions to differentiate are intraparotid Kaposi's sarcoma (Fig. 78) and lymphoma, although infections such as MAI may also involve salivary tissue.

Management Fine-needle aspiration reduces the size of the mass, but may need to be repeated. It also provides material for cytology and culture. Neoplastic and infectious pathology should be managed as outlined elsewhere. Cystic change does not require specific treatment.

Xerostomia

Dryness of the mouth complicates 5–10% of AIDS cases. The aetiology is unknown, but chronic HIV sialadenitis probably plays a part. Specific treatment with synthetic saliva is occasionally required.

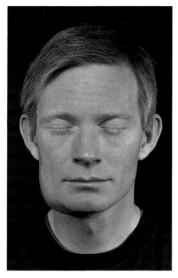

Fig. 77 Unilateral parotid enlargement in a 40-year-old man with AIDS.

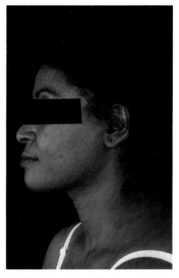

Fig. 78 Left parotid swelling due to Kaposi's sarcoma.

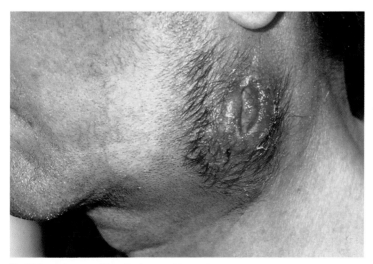

Fig. 79 Fungating wound 3 weeks after open biopsy of a neck mass. This proved to be lymphoma.

16 / Cervical lymphadenopathy

The commonest cause in HIV infection is PGL (p. 11), but the important differentials require description.

Differential diagnosis

Lymphoma. This is a common site for lymphoma to present. Unilateral, rapidly progressive nodal enlargement may be superimposed on PGL or occur 'de novo' (Figs 80 & 81). Constitutional symptoms, such as night sweats are common.

Kaposi's sarcoma may spread to regional nodes.

Squamous cell carcinoma of the head and neck commonly metastasizes to cervical nodes. A primary site in the head and neck should be sought

Mycobacterial infection. In AIDS, *MAI* is commoner than *M.tuberculosis*, and may occur even in the absence of chest disease (Fig. 49, p. 42).

Investigations

Full blood count may suggest infection, while skin tests may support a diagnosis of mycobacterial involvement. Fine-needle aspiration cytology is preferred to open biopsy of neck nodes, as only 10% of open biopsies uncover substantial pathology, and HIV patients heal poorly. Nevertheless, if suspicion of lymphoma remains, open biopsy becomes necessary (Fig. 79, p. 64).

Management

This depends on the underlying cause. Mycobacterial infections may recur.

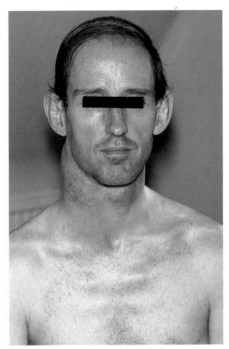

Fig. 80 Unilateral cervical lymphadenopathy: non-Hodgkins lymphoma.

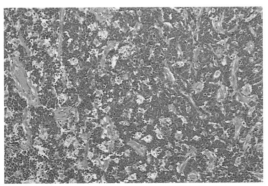

Fig. 81 'Starry sky' histological appearance of AIDS-related non-Hodgkin's lymphoma. .

17 / **Gastrointestinal tract**

Oesophageal candidiasis

This is the commonest opportunistic infection of the GIT and is an indicator disease for AIDS. The distal oesophagus is the most frequent site.

Pathology

Most infections are by *C.albicans*, although *C.glabrata* may also occur. The pseudomembranous form, consisting of invasive hyphae with surrounding necrosis, is commoner than the exophytic form. Pseudohyphae do not extend beyond the serosa.

Clinical features

Patients present with retrosternal chest pain and painful dysphagia, or may be asymptomatic. Associated oral candidiasis is common. Like other causes of longstanding chronic inflammation, candidiasis can cause strictures.

Diagnosis

This can be established by barium swallow (Fig. 82) or on endoscopy (Fig. 83). Biopsy or brushings for cytology should be taken to look for invasive pseudohyphae. Culture is not very useful because of the ubiquity of candida.

Differential diagnosis

Similar symptoms can result from other opportunistic infections, e.g. herpes, *MAI*, ulcerating hairy leukoplakia or neoplasia, any of which may coexist.

Management

Oral antifungal agents, e.g. ketoconazole, are required. Topical treatment with, for example, amphoterocin lozenges may supplement this. Maintenance therapy is necessary.

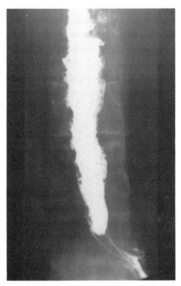

Fig. 82 Barium swallow in oesophageal candidiasis: irregular outline due to swelling and oedema.

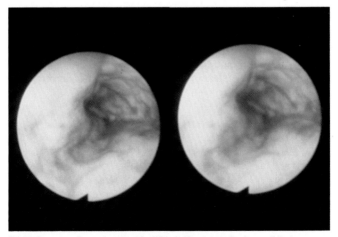

Fig. 83 Severe confluent oesophagitis visible at 23 cm proved to be candidiasis.

Cytomegalovirus (CMV)

Primary infection with this herpes virus is common in homosexuals and intravenous drug users. Repeated reactivation, shown by reappearance of anti-CMV-IgM, occurs during HIV infection and may cause disease at any point along the GIT.

CMV oesophagitis

Pathology
Infection commences in submucosal cells, where inclusion bodies may be seen. Serpiginous ulcers are characteristic (Figs 84 & 85).

Clinical features
Antifungal-resistant, severe odynophagia is typical. Other evidence of CMV disease, e.g. colitis, may be present.

Diagnosis
The non-specific nature of barium swallow renders endoscopy and biopsy with viral cultures essential.

Management
Virostatic agents (ganciclovir, foscarnet) may lead to long-term remission. Maintenance therapy is not always necessary.

CMV colitis

Clinical features
Up to 10% of AIDS cases are complicated by this. Profuse, liquid diarrhoea, up to 20 stools per day, is characteristic and abdominal pain and weight loss are usual. Rectal bleeding, perforation and toxic dilatation all occur and may be fatal. Untreated, chronic symptoms occur unless punctuated by abdominal catastrophe.

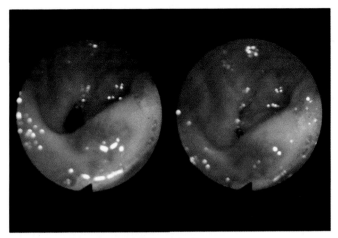

Fig. 84 Endoscopic appearances of CMV oesophagitis.

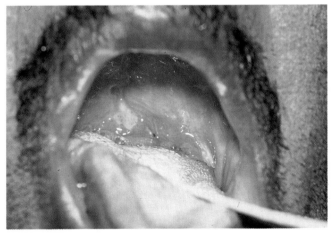

Fig. 85 Serpiginous ulcers of the oropharynx in a patient with CMV oesophagitis.

Differential diagnosis	Other infecting organisms, e.g. *Shigella, Clostridium difficile* or *MAI*, and inflammatory bowel disease may all present in similar fashion to CMV colitis.
Diagnosis	Having excluded other infectious causes by multiple stool cultures, sigmoidoscopy with rectal biopsy should be performed. Colonoscopy or flexible sigmoidoscopy is rarely required as involvement of the rectum is almost invariable (Fig. 86).
Management	Acutely, parenteral fluids and nutrition are required. Treatment is with ganciclovir/foscarnet.

Herpes simplex virus (HSV)

Since most adults with AIDS have been infected with HSV types I and/or II, reactivation is common and may affect various parts of the GIT.

Herpes simplex oesophagitis

Pathology	HSV causes epithelial necrosis. The early vesicles slough, causing circumscribed ulcers (Fig. 87).
Clinical features	Characteristically, there is painful dysphagia. There may be associated pharyngeal ulceration.
Diagnosis	Endoscopic biopsy for histological demonstration of invasive viral infection and viral culture is necessary.
Management	High-dose intravenous acyclovir is required, followed by maintenance oral therapy.

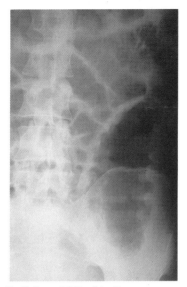

Fig. 86 X-ray of CMV colitis with 'thumbprinting' and thickening of bowel wall due to oedema.

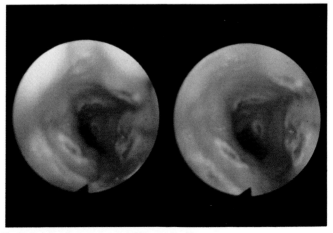

Fig. 87 Endoscopic appearances of HSV oesophagitis.

Cryptosporidiosis

Pathology   Infection with the protozoan, *Cryptosporidium parvum* causes mild symptoms in the immunocompetent, but in AIDS it persists and can be progressively fatal. It affects any portion of the GIT, particularly the small bowel and biliary tree (10%). Enterocyte infection causes villous fusion.

Clinical features   Severe watery diarrhoea and anorexia are usual. Vomiting and nausea characterize biliary involvement. Episodes last for weeks or months.

Diagnosis   Acid-fast staining demonstrates cysts of *C.parvum* in stool specimens (Fig. 88).

Management   Despite trials of various drugs, there is no satisfactory treatment. Oral rehydration solutions and nutritional supplements are useful, and symptomatic relief of diarrhoea, vomiting and abdominal pain should be attempted. There have been recent reports of symptomatic relief with Paromomycin and Sandostatin (somatostatin analogue).

Mycobacterial infection

Pathology   *Mycobacterium avium intracellulare* affects the GIT as part of disseminated disease. Acid-fast organisms are found in stools or biopsies (Fig. 89).

Clinical features   Presentation is with fever, night sweats, periumbilical pain and diarrhoea.

Management   Symptomatic relief with combination chemotherapy may be achieved, but eradication is difficult.

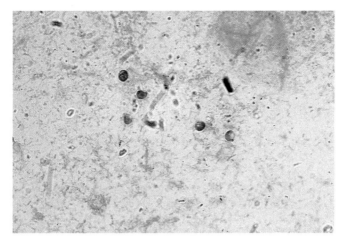

Fig. 88 Cysts of *Cryptosporidium parvum* in stool specimen.

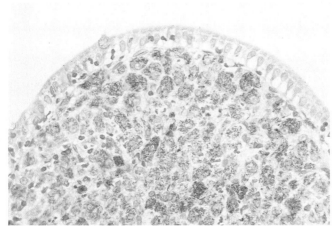

Fig. 89 Small intestinal biopsy showing lamina propria histiocytes and numerous atypical AAFBs.

Kaposi's sarcoma

Clinical features Visceral or intestinal KS is usually asymptomatic but may give rise to perforation, obstruction or haemorrhage. Jaundice may result from biliary obstruction. Protein-losing enteropathy due to mesenteric lymphatic obstruction is described.

Diagnosis Filling defects occur on barium studies (Fig. 90). Flat or polypoid, purple lesions are seen on endoscopy (Fig. 91). Biopsy features are similar to those of KS elsewhere (Fig. 36, p. 32).

Management Intestinal KS only requires treatment if symptomatic. Combination chemotherapy followed by maintenance single or alternating agents may be tried, but immunosuppression may be problematic.

Lymphoma

Clinical features The GIT is the commonest site for extranodal lymphoma in AIDS. Presentation depends on the site:
- dysphagia and chest pain in oesophagus
- haematemesis in gastric disease (Fig. 92)
- obstruction, perforation or intussusception (Fig. 93) with bowel tumours
- altered bowel habit and bleeding with rectal lesions
- hepatic and nodal masses are often asymptomatic.

Fever and night sweats are non-specific features.

Diagnosis Localization with various imaging techniques must be followed by histological confirmation (Fig. 81, p. 66). Fine-needle biopsy, ascitic aspiration, peritoneoscopy or laparotomy all play a role.

Prognosis Median survival is 6 months even with chemotherapy.

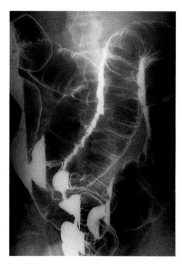

Fig. 90 Barium enema showing irregular mucosa and some narrowing of the sigmoid and rectum: KS.

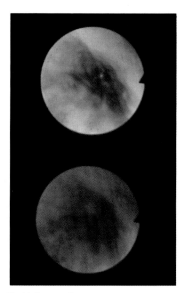

Fig. 91 Scattered bluish lesions of the duodenum consistent with Kaposi's sarcoma.

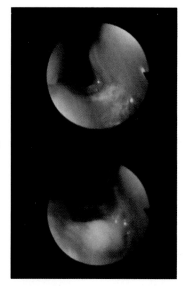

Fig. 92 Endoscopic appearances of ulcerated gastric lymphoma.

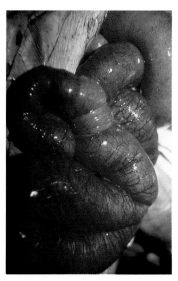

Fig. 93 Operative picture demonstrating ileal intussusception due to lymphoma.

18 / Genitourinary medicine

Patients with HIV infection should be offered screening for other sexually transmitted diseases (STDs). Genital ulceration in particular affects morbidity and the transmission of HIV (p. 107).

Genital herpes (HSV)

Pathology

Primary infection with HSV usually predates that with HIV. Both HSV I and II are seen. Acquisition is by contact of broken skin or mucous membranes with sercretions or mucous membranes of a carrier (Fig. 94). The virus ascends via peripheral nerves, to establish latency within the ganglia.

Clinical features

Primary genital herpes is characterized by multiple, painful vesicles which may coalesce and ulcerate. Symptoms include dysuria, discharge due to cervicitis, and rectal discharge and tenesmus due to proctitis. Inguinal lymphadenopathy and systemic symptoms of fever, aches and pains may coexist. Episodes last about 2 weeks, but immunosuppression may prolong the episode or encourage dissemination.

Recurrent HSV presents as parasthesiae and pain, with vesicles and ulcers (Fig. 95). In AIDS, recurrences increase in frequency and may last for weeks.

Management

Primary disease. Confirmation is by viral culture of vesicle or ulcer fluid. Standard doses of acyclovir may need to be increased in immunosuppression.

Recurrent disease. Maintenance acyclovir therapy is recommended for all patients with HIV suffering recurrences.

Disseminated disease requires high-dose parenteral therapy. Foscarnet is an alternative in resistant cases.

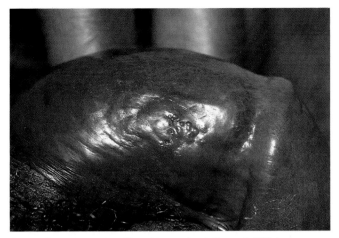

Fig. 94 HSV type I was cultured from this case of genital herpes in HIV infection.

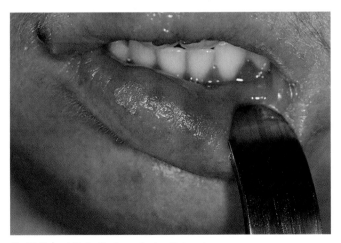

Fig. 95 Herpes labialis affecting perioral and intraoral areas.

Anogenital warts

Aetiology Genital warts are caused by infection of the epidermis by human papilloma virus (HPV), which is usually sexually transmitted.

Pathology Genital warts are pleomorphic. Exophytic warts (condylomata acuminata) are commonest, but papular or flat forms and the common wart (verruca vulgaris) may occur. There is an epidemiological association between women with cytological evidence of HPV and cervical dysplasia. It is unclear as to whether this association is greater in the presence of HIV disease.

Clinical features The commonest sites are the subpreputial area in men (Fig. 96) and the fourchette in women (Fig. 97). They also occur commonly in the urethral meatus, perineum, in the anal canal (Fig. 97) and on the vagina and cervix. Warts may also occur at extragenital sites, such as the mouth and the nipple. Genital warts tend to be more extensive and resistant to therapy in HIV infection.

Management There are three main modalities of treatment:
- *Cytotoxic agents* such as podophyllin, 5-fluoro-uracil and topical trichloroacetic acid (TCAA).
- *Surgery* by cryotherapy, electrocautery, diathermy, or laser.
- *Immune-modulating agents* such as interferon.

Of these, podophyllin and cryotherapy are most commonly used, but intra-anal warts often require excision (Fig. 96).

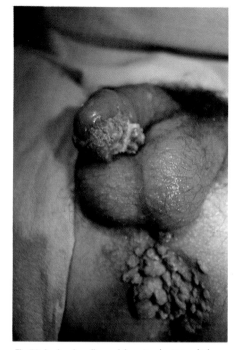

Fig. 96 Anal and penile condylomata prior to surgical excision.

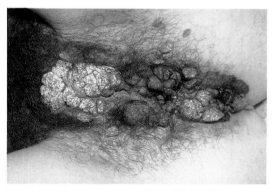

Fig. 97 Anogenital warts involving perineum and extending into anal and vaginal canals.

Vulvovaginal and anorectal candidiasis

Aetiology   This is caused mainly by *Candida albicans*, which is a commensal in the gastrointestinal tract where it may become invasive due to impaired mucosal immunity (Fig. 3). A similar event may underlie vaginal candidiasis (thrush). Infection may spread from the anus. Perianal candidiasis is rare in the general population, but common in HIV infection.

Clinical features   Patients present with pruritus and vaginal discharge. There may be local pain, external dysuria and superficial dyspareunia. On examination, there is vulval oedema with surrounding inflammation, vaginal mucosal erythema or superficial erosions. The discharge is classically likened to 'cottage-cheese' (Fig. 98), but it may also be thin, homogenous or scanty. The appearance of perianal disease is similar, with intertrigo possibly extending between the buttocks (Fig. 99).

Differential diagnosis   Vaginitis due to *Trichomonas vaginalis* (TV) and bacterial vaginosis may be excluded by examining a direct smear from the posterior fornix under dark ground microscopy. Spores or hyphae may be visualized by Gram-staining, or by examining scrapings from intertriginous areas. Culture is possible from vaginal or anal swabs.

Management   For vaginal and rectal disease, creams or pessaries (e.g. nystatin) are used. For intertrigo, topical preparations are effective. Oral agents, e.g. ketoconazole, are used in resistant cases or as prophylaxis against oesophageal candidiasis.

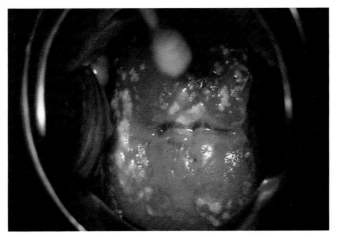

Fig. 98 Vulvovaginal candidiasis: white plaques of candida are adherent to the cervix.

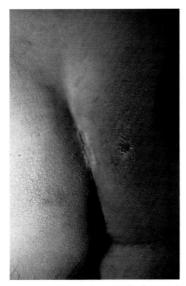

Fig. 99 Perianal intertrigo extending into natal cleft. There is also a buttock abscess.

Gonorrhoea

Incidence Statistics for new cases of gonorrhoea dropped rapidly at the onset of the AIDS epidemic, but recent reports show a slight rise.

Clinical features Gonorrhoea may be asymptomatic, especially in female patients. Urethral (Fig. 100), rectal, pharyngeal, cervical and disseminated gonorrhoea have been reported in AIDS, with site-specific symptoms. Treatment is with conventional antibiotics.

Syphilis

Primary infection is rarely seen in HIV infection in developed countries. However, there remains a firm association between positive syphilis serology and HIV. HIV may alter the natural history of syphilis: there is earlier neurological involvement and penicillin treatment may be less effective (Fig. 101).

Other anogenital conditions

STDs sometimes seen include hepatitis B, chancroid, lymphogranuloma venereum and scabies. Kaposi's sarcoma is seen on genital skin and mucous membranes and may produce inguinal lymphadenopathy (Fig. 102). Male homosexuals with HIV infection are particularly prone to infected perianal conditions (Fig. 103).

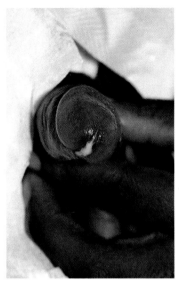

Fig. 100 Urethral discharge of gonococcal infection.

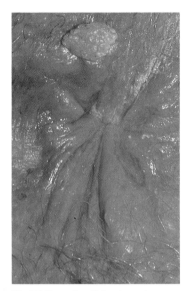

Fig. 101 Unusual multiple primary chancres of syphilis in the perianal area. Note also genital warts.

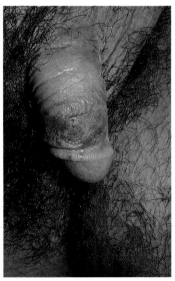

Fig. 102 Purplish patch of Kaposi's sarcoma on penis.

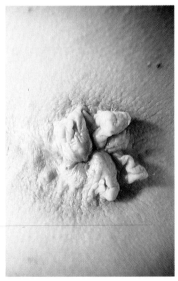

Fig. 103 Pruritic perianal skin tags in a man with HIV infection.

19 / **Primary neurological disease**

Neurological complications affect 39% of patients with AIDS, although nervous involvement at postmortem is nearer 90%. It is now well-recognized that the HIV is neurotropic as well as lymphotropic, so that a large part of neurological manifestations are a direct result of HIV infection. Opportunistic infection of the central nervous system (CNS) is also common and is considered below.

Subacute encephalitis

Incidence This is the commonest neurological manifestation of HIV infection. Without treatment about a third of patients with AIDS eventually develop a form of this disease.

Pathology Brain cultures from these patients have revealed a mixture of pathologies, especially CMV infection. However, the high correlation of this condition with HIV-1 p24 antigen in the CSF, and the presence of HIV inclusion bodies on brain biopsy indicate that this is a primary manifestation of the HIV itself. Histologically, encephalitis is characterized by the presence of giant cells (Fig. 104).

Clinical features **AIDS dementia syndrome.** This is characterized by a progressive confusional state with occasional frontal lobe signs. Mild headache is common.
Focal deficit such as hemianopia may occur.

Investigations Psychological testing reveals cognitive deficits of varying severity. CSF protein is raised, whilst CT and MRI scans are usually normal until the late stages, when cortical atrophy becomes evident (Fig. 105).

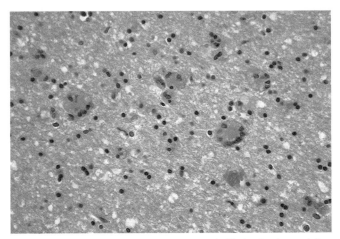

Fig. 104 Brain biopsy from a patient with subacute encephalitis showing characteristic giant cells.

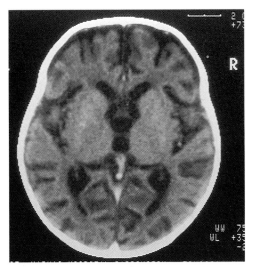

Fig. 105 CT scan of a patient with AIDS dementia syndrome with enlarged sulci of cortical atrophy.

Management   Apart from psychological support for the patient and relatives, there is no specific treatment for subacute encephalitis. However, its appearance or progression may be delayed by the introduction of zidovudine.

Atypical aseptic meningitis

This has a similar pathological appearance to subacute encephalitis. As this occurs at the onset of HIV infection (p. 9), the different presentation may reflect different levels of immune competence.

Clinical features   Episodes of meningism with variable focal signs, especially cranial nerve palsies, which tend to recur. CSF shows pleocytosis and raised protein.

Myelopathy

Pathology   Patients may present with long tract signs. Histology in these cases shows vacuoles containing macrophages (Fig. 106).

Neuropathy

Clinical features   **Cranial neuropathy.** This is commonly found in association with infections: meningitis, toxoplasmosis and herpes zoster. Cerebral lymphoma may present with cranial nerve lesions, whilst Bell's palsy (Fig. 107) is also common.

Chronic polyneuropathy. The commonest form is painful sensory neuropathy (Fig. 108). Inflammatory neuropathy has been reported in the US.

Guillain–Barré-type syndrome. This is thought to be an autoimmune-mediated aspect of HIV infection.

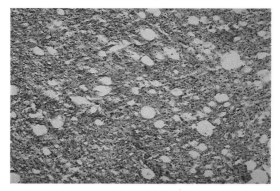

Fig. 106 Vacuolar myelopathy in a patient with lower limb weakness.

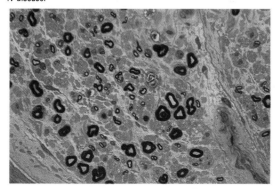

Fig. 107 Left facial weakness due to Bell's palsy in a man with stage IV disease.

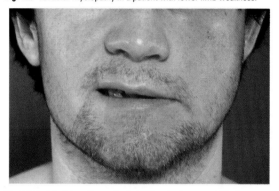

Fig. 108 Sural nerve biopsy in sensory neuropathy: decreased myelinated fibres, some degenerate.

20 / Opportunistic infections of the CNS

These are common in AIDS. It is important to remember that such infections sometimes coexist with each other and with other pathologies.

Toxoplasma gondii

Toxoplasmosis is one of the commonest of human infections, with seropositivity ranging from 20–70% in the US, and is associated with ingestion of meat. Infection is often subclinical in healthy individuals, but reactivation in HIV infection can be life-threatening.

Pathology Acute focal or diffuse meningoencephalitis with cellular necrosis associated with intra- and extra-cellular trophozoites is seen (Figs 109 & 110). Necrotizing granulomas with little inflammation are characteristic. Thrombosis of blood vessels causing large areas of coagulation necrosis may produce mass lesions (Fig. 111).

Clinical features Initial symptoms are headache and lethargy followed by focal signs. Untreated, seizures, confusion and impaired conscious level ensue. The condition may be fatal.

Investigations **Serological tests** are unreliable, although toxoplasma antibody is usually present.

CT or MRI scans may reveal focal abnormality or may be normal. Where there is reasonable suspicion, empirical treatment should be instituted. Definitive diagnosis rests on brain biopsy.

Management Six weeks of pyrimethamine and sulphadiazine are used, with indefinite maintenance therapy. Response may be followed by repeat CT/MRI scans.

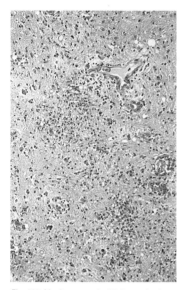

Fig. 109 Meningoencephalitis in cerebral toxoplasmosis: trophozoites and weak inflammatory response.

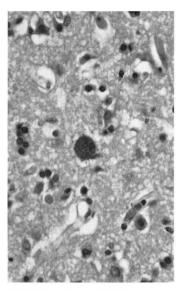

Fig. 110 Biopsy from a frontal lobe pseudocyst. Toxoplasma trophozoite is seen centrally.

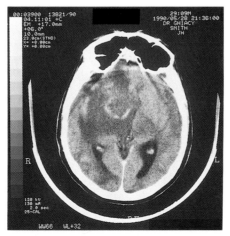

Fig. 111 CT scan in toxoplasmosis: ring-enhancing lesion with surrounding oedema and mass effect.

Cryptococcus neoformans

This is the commonest fungal infection of the CNS. Route of infection is via the respiratory tract.

Clinical features Patients with cryptococcal meningitis present with headache, sometimes associated with confusion, focal signs (Fig. 112) or seizures. CT and MRI scans are usually normal but may show cerebral atrophy or hydrocephalus (Fig. 113).

Investigations India ink preparations (Fig. 114) of CSF give rapid diagnosis, then confirmed by culture. Latex agglutination for cryptococcal antigen is positive in meningitis.

Management Therapy is with amphoterocin B and 5-flucytosine. Recurrences occur despite maintenance therapy. Overall mortality is high.

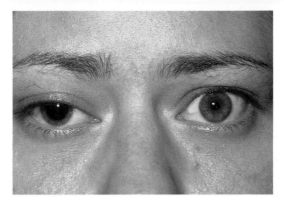

Fig. 112 Right third nerve palsy in a patient with cryptococcal meningitis.

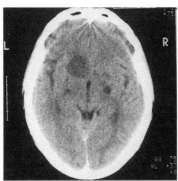

Fig. 113 Cerebral cryptococcoma: low attenuation lesion initially treated as toxoplasma.

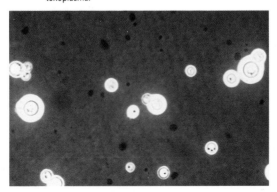

Fig. 114 *Cryptococcus neoformans* demonstrated by India ink preparation of CSF from an obtunded patient.

Progressive multifocal leukoencephalopathy (PML)

Clinical features This demyelinating condition presents with progressive mental aberrations, blindness, aphasias, hemiparesis and other focal deficits. CT or MRI scans (Fig. 115) show non-enhancing white matter lesions without mass effect or oedema.

Pathology Brain biopsy shows focal myelin loss with an absence of inflammation and enlarged, pleomorphic oligodendrocytes containing eosinophilic viral inclusion bodies (Fig. 116), thought to represent CMV infection.

Prognosis Cytosine arabinoside has been reported to help. However, most cases progress slowly to death.

Other infections

Mycobacteria. Both *M.tuberculosis* and *M.avium intracellulare* have been described in HIV infection, causing meningitis and tuberculoma.

Candida albicans can extend to the CNS, usually in cases of disseminated candidiasis.

Coccidiodomycosis is a persistent problem in HIV patients in the Southwestern US in particular. Most present with a chronic relapsing meningitis.

Bacteria are infrequently involved in infections of the CNS in HIV patients.

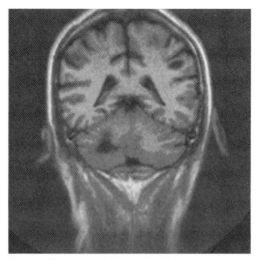

Fig. 115 MRI scan in PML with typical patchy lesions.

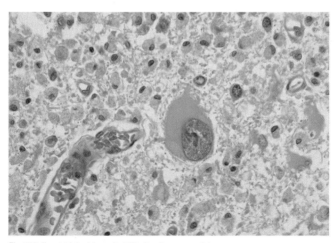

Fig. 116 Frontal lobe biopsy in PML showing areas of demyelination and an absence of inflammation.

21 / CNS neoplasia

Primary cerebral lymphoma

Pathology These are large cell lymphomas similar to those previously seen in other immunosuppressed states.

Clinical features Presentation may be with encephalopathy, brain-stem abnormality or cranial neuropathy. CSF is often normal, but may contain elevated protein or atypical cells. CT or MRI scans demonstrate hypodense areas with peripheral enhancement (Fig. 117).

Differential diagnosis Other space-occupying lesions, especially infections such as toxoplasmosis and other neoplasias. Where doubt exists, brain biopsy under stereotactic guidance is indicated.

Management Radiotherapy and chemotherapy may slow the progress, but most are rapidly fatal.

Other tumours

Systemic lymphoma involving the CNS may occur, and especially affects the meninges, causing cranial neuropathy.

Kaposi's Sarcoma may spread to the brain.

Myositis

Painful inflammatory myositis has been described in connection with HIV infection. This may be an autoimmune phenomenon, although viral inclusion bodies are sometimes seen on biopsy.

Myopathy

The commonest myopathy seen in AIDS is that related to zidovudine therapy (Figs 118 & 119). A condition similar to motor neurone disease has also been described.

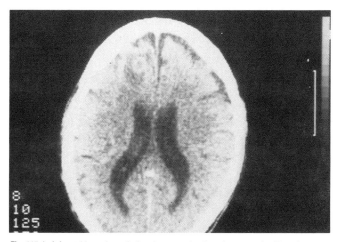

Fig. 117 Left frontal hypodense lesion that proved to be primary cerebral lymphoma on brain biopsy.

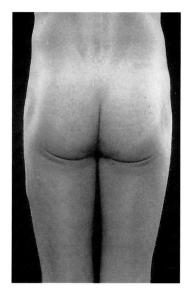

Fig. 118 Wasting of gluteal and quadriceps muscles in zidovudine-related proximal myopathy.

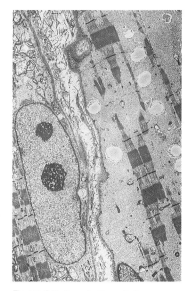

Fig. 119 EM of muscle biopsy in the same patient in Figure 118, showing atrophy and abnormal mitochondria.

As many as 65% of AIDS patients are reported to have ocular pathology at some time. Of these, by far the commonest are cotton wool spots and CMV retinitis.

Cytomegalovirus (CMV) retinitis

Clinical features   Patients present with floaters or visual loss, or may be diagnosed on routine screening. The involved eyes are not painful or red. There may be visual field defects with absolute scotomas. Fundoscopic findings are variable (Figs 120 & 121).

Management   Ganciclovir, an inhibitor of viral DNA polymerase, is the treatment of choice. A two-week intravenous induction course is followed by maintenance therapy, possibly self-injecting via a Hickman line. Foscarnet may be used alone if side-effects (neutropenia, thrombocytopenia, neuropathy) prove troublesome, or in combination.

Prognosis   Untreated, progression to bilateral blindness within six months is usual. Death may be from another opportunistic infection or malignancy, or from multisystem CMV involvement.

Other opportunistic ocular infections

Ocular toxoplasmosis, choroidal cryptococcosis, *Pneumocystis carinii* retinitis and choroidal mycobacterial granulomata have been described but are less common. Retinal haemorrhage may occur in zidovudine-related anaemia (p. 113). It resolves with transfusion.

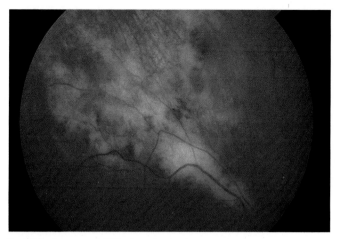

Fig. 120 Early, segmental CMV retinopathy showing areas of exudation and haemorrhage.

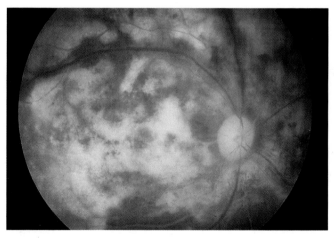

Fig. 121 Atrophic retina following CMV retinitis.

Cotton wool spots

Clinical features   These are superficial white retinal opacities that tend to spontaneously regress over a period of a few weeks (Fig. 122). They are thought to represent areas of ischaemia in the retinal nerve fibre layer and are not associated with any visual loss. Cotton wool spots tend to regress and recur during the course of HIV disease.

Differential diagnosis   Cotton wool spots may precede the development of overt CMV retinitis. It is therefore essential to perform serial observations. Other conditions causing cotton wool spots, such as diabetes, hypertension and collagen vascular disease are uncommonly found in HIV infection.

Conjunctival Kaposi's sarcoma

Clinical features   These may occur on any part of the conjunctiva, and are rarely large enough to cause visual disturbance (Fig. 123).

Differential diagnosis   Misdiagnosis of the lesions as haemorrhage or haemangioma is possible.

Management   If the lesions threaten vision or are cosmetically unacceptable, local excision or radiotherapy may be considered.

Ocular motility disorders

Clinical features   These may affect cranial nerves III, IV or VI. In all cases, the possibility of intracranial pathology such as toxoplasmosis, cryptococcosis or lymphoma should be excluded (pp. 89–96, and Fig. 112).

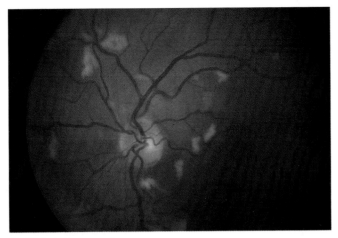

Fig. 122 Retinal cotton-wool spots.

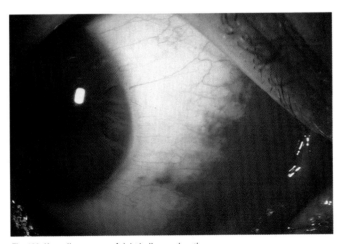

Fig. 123 Kaposi's sarcoma of right bulbar conjunctiva.

23 / **Paediatric AIDS**

Aetiology Transmission to infants and children is mainly vertical, about 1 in 5 children born to HIV infected mothers being infected. Currently, half of European cases were transmitted by infected blood products. Transmission via maternal milk is also possible.

Incidence A WHO estimate suggests that there may be 10 million children infected with HIV by the year 2000. AIDS may thus become a major cause of infant mortality worldwide.

Early signs

Clinical features Failure to thrive and weight loss (Fig. 124), recurrent diarrhoea, protein-losing enteropathy (Fig. 125), poor hair growth, dermatitis and PGL are all common presenting features.

Diagnosis The appearance of the above features in an at-risk child merits careful investigation. Other causes of failure to thrive and immunosuppression should be specifically excluded. Maternal antibodies may persist for up to 18 months in these children, making HIV antibody testing unreliable before this age. Persistent hypergammaglobulinaemia may be used as a marker in these patients. More specific tests are being developed but are not yet widely available.

Prognosis The recent European Collaborative Study suggests that 48% of infected children show clinical signs by 6 months; 26% have AIDS and 17% die of HIV-related disease by 12 months. Progression appears to be slower after this.

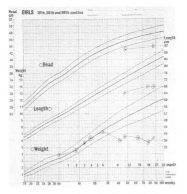

Fig. 124 Progress chart showing decline from 50th centile at six months.

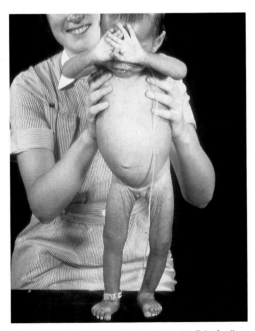

Fig. 125 A child of two years with failure-to-thrive. Tube-feeding due to oral thrush.

Opportunistic infections

Bacteria. Unlike adults, children with HIV infection may have had no opportunity to form antibodies to common bacteria, and so suffer from increased bacterial and mycobacterial infections, such as otitis media, pneumonia and meningitis.

Viruses. Similarly, these children are particularly vulnerable to the common viral infections of childhood, such as varicella–zoster. Viral infections prevalent in adults with AIDS are also seen, particularly herpes simplex (Fig. 126) and cytomegalovirus.

Fungi. Candidal infection is common, and may present as a severe form of nappy-rash (Fig. 127), oral thrush or oesophageal disease (Fig. 128).

Pneumocystis carinii pneumonia (PCP)

As with adult disease, this is a major complication in paediatric AIDS, often contributing to death.

Clinical features Children may present with unproductive cough and malaise. CXR (Fig. 129, p. 106) is very variable and diagnosis may require lung biopsy or BAL (p. 39).

Management As in adults with low CD4 counts, prophylactic treatment with cotrimoxazole should be instituted.

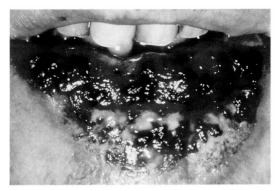

Fig. 126 Severe herpes simplex of lower lip in paediatric AIDS.

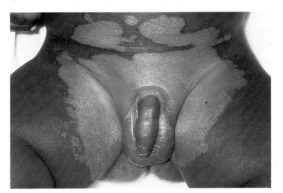

Fig. 127 Scarring following severe candidal nappy rash.

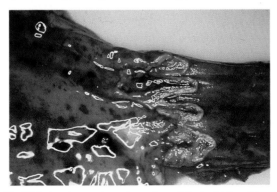

Fig. 128 Postmortem specimen of oesophagus following fatal candida-related perforation.

Lymphocytic interstitial pneumonitis (LIP)

Many HIV-infected children develop this condition in which there is extensive lymphoid infiltration of the lung, leading to a restrictive picture.

Clinical features Failure-to-thrive is common, with progressive compromise of respiratory function. CXR shows diffuse bilateral reticulonodular infiltrates and sometimes hilar lymphadenopathy (Fig. 131).

Management There are anecdotal reports of benefit from zidovudine in symptomatic cases.

Neurological disorders

In addition to developmental delay, acquired microcephaly, seizures and encephalopathy occur. At postmortem, there is often calcification of vessels in basal ganglia, and white matter atrophy.

Other features

Lymphadenopathy and hepatosplenomegaly are often found at presentation, and bilateral parotid enlargement (Fig. 130) may be seen. Unlike in adults, malignancy is rare in HIV-infected children.

General management of paediatric AIDS

Children with HIV infection require vigorous nutritional support. Intravenous immunoglobulin may reduce the frequency of bacterial infections but a beneficial effect on survival has not yet been demonstrated. The place of zidovudine in paediatric HIV-infection awaits confirmation, but it should probably be given in advanced disease. Careful psychological and social support is necessary for the child and his family.

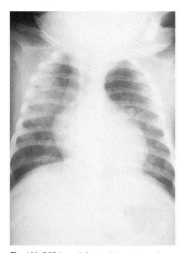

Fig. 129 PCP in an infant, with patches of consolidation in the right upper zone.

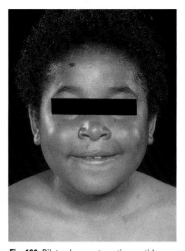

Fig. 130 Bilateral asymptomatic parotid enlargement in a child with LIP.

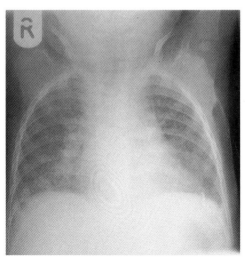

Fig. 131 LIP with diffuse bilateral reticulonodular infiltrate and hilar lymphadenopathy.

24 / **HIV infection in Africa**

It has been speculated that AIDS has its origins in a remote region of Africa, possibly the Belgian Congo (now Zaire). However, the current rate of spread of the disease in Sub-Saharan Africa suggests that it is, even there, a new disease.

Incidence   The absence of organized data collection from most areas of Africa means that any figures are likely to be inaccurate and are probably underestimates. However, best estimates of distribution (Fig. 1, p. 2, and Fig. 132) indicate that 1 in 40 people in urban areas of Central Africa is HIV-positive. In Abidjan, it is the leading cause of mortality in men and second only to perinatal deaths in women. Unlike Western patterns, sex distribution is about equal, and vertical transmission to children is more likely (30% chance).

Aetiology   Contrasted with Western AIDS, the most striking aspect of the African form is the predominance of heterosexual transmission. Central to this is the economic and social dependence of the woman on sexual relations with men. In this setting, sexually-transmitted disease is common and consequent genital ulceration predisposes to transmission of HIV. Prostitution is also a factor, as is the lack of barrier contraception. The use of increased blood transfusions also increases the risk. HIV-2 also leads to disease, but progression may be slower.

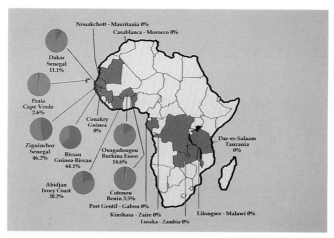

Fig. 132 Distribution of HIV-2 in Africa. The pie charts show the proportions of population infected in specific areas.

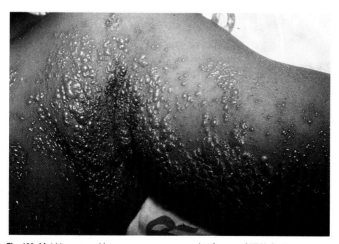

Fig. 133 Multidermatomal herpes zoster as a presenting feature of HIV infection.

Diarrhoea ('slim disease')

Aetiology Wasting related to diarrhoea is a common feature of African HIV infection, and is locally termed 'Slim Disease'. *Cryptosporidium* and *Isospora belli* are identified in up to 60% of cases, but it is unclear whether they are the causes of the diarrhoea.

Clinical features Intermittent, chronic diarrhoea in a previously fit adult, causing marked weight loss in most cases.

Herpes zoster

Clinical features This is frequently the first clinical presentation and has a positive predictive value for HIV positivity of 95%. It may be protracted and multidermatomal (Fig. 133, p. 108).

Tuberculosis (TB)

Incidence This is the most common opportunistic infection associated with African AIDS. About 60% of all persons with tuberculosis are HIV-positive, rising to 80% for those with pleural and pericardial disease. Extrapulmonary tuberculosis is also more common in HIV-positive individuals.

Aetiology In a community where both HIV and tuberculosis are endemic, AIDS tuberculosis may represent a new infection or reactivation.

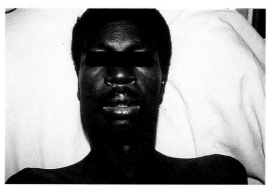

Fig. 134 Bilateral cervical lymphadenopathy due to tuberculosis.

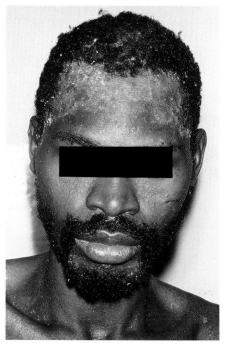

Fig. 135 Psoriasis in an African man who also had pulmonary tuberculosis.

Clinical features Pulmonary TB in HIV-infected patients is less likely to be associated with positive sputum smears. Chest X-rays are usually abnormal compared to HIV-negative subjects, but less often show the upper zone disease of 'classical' tuberculosis. Extrapulmonary, especially nodal, disease (Fig. 134, p. 110) is common. Other HIV-related conditions often coexist (Fig. 135, p. 110).

Prognosis The course of the disease, even when triple therapy is available, is protracted and tuberculosis is the leading cause of AIDS-related deaths in Africa.

Other opportunistic infections

These are determined by environmental exposure. Thus, *Pneumocystis carinii* pneumonia is uncommon, whilst leishmaniasis, toxoplasmosis, salmonellosis and cryptococcal meningitis are all well-recognized.

Kaposi's sarcoma

AIDS–KS coexists in Africa with an endemic form, from which it differs clinically.

Clinical features Compared with endemic disease, there are more patch and plaque lesions, and a smaller proportion of nodular lesions (Figs 136 & 137). Visceral disease is much more common. Histologically, lesions have less inflammation. African AIDS–KS may be more aggressive than that seen in developed countries.

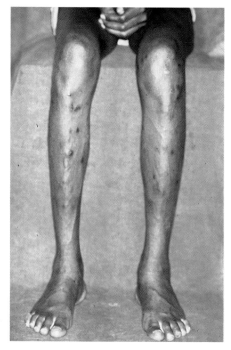

Fig. 136 Multiple plaque and nodular lesions of Kaposi's sarcoma.

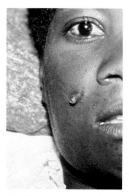

Fig. 137 Facial and conjunctival KS in an African woman with AIDS.

25 / Approaches to therapy

Zidovudine

Mechanism
Zidovudine (AZT) is the only specific anti-HIV agent currently licensed for use. It is a nucleoside analogue and inhibits reverse transcriptase (Fig. 138).

Indications
Originally it was only used in patients with an AIDS-defining diagnosis or AIDS-related complex. The Federal Drugs Advisory Board (FDA) in the USA now recommends initiation of therapy in any HIV-positive patient who has 2 consecutive CD4 cell counts (6 weeks apart) less than 500. However, these guidelines are not universally applied.

Clinical application
Multicentre studies have shown that zidovudine improves survival and quality of life in patients with AIDS and reduces the frequency and severity of opportunistic infections. Maintenance dose is currently 500 mg/d.

Complications
In the first weeks of therapy, headache, nausea and malaise may occur. The complications of long-term therapy have restricted its use. Marrow suppression (Fig. 139) manifests itself as anaemia about 3 months after commencement in 1–30% of patients, depending on dose and stage of disease. A proximal myopathy (Fig. 118, p. 96) associated with a rise in creatin kinase tends to resolve on withdrawal of the drug. Nail hyperpigmentation (Fig. 140, p. 116) is also seen on long-term zidovudine.

Other reverse transcriptase inhibitors

These include the following:

- *Dideoxyinosine* (DDI) is in an advanced stage of testing, employing patients intolerant of zidovudine. Side-effects are vomiting, pancreatitis and peripheral neuropathy.
- *Dideoxycytidine* (DDC) is also under trial.
- *Phosphonofornate*.
- *R82913*.

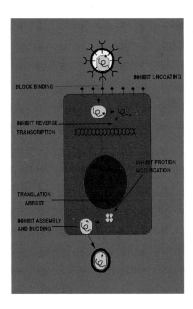

Fig. 138 The life-cycle of HIV showing potential sites for therapeutic modulation.

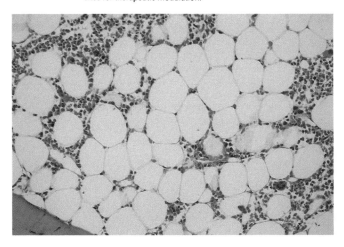

Fig. 139 Hypocellular bone-marrow trephine from a patient with AZT-related myelosuppression.

Other agents

Other agents used in HIV therapy include the following:
- *Protease inhibitors* act against viral assembly.
- *Alpha-interferon* operates at a number of sites.
- *Soluble CD4* competitively antagonizes the binding of HIV to host CD4 lymphocytes (Fig. 138, p. 114).

Long-term antiviral treatment

Long-term therapy may sometimes require the siting of central lines, and this facilitates treatment at home (Fig. 141).

Future trends in HIV infection

In the 10 years since the first case of AIDS was reported, the median survival time after an AIDS diagnosis has gone from under 6 months to around 2 years. Reasons for this include earlier diagnosis of HIV infection, antiretroviral treatment and prophylaxis against and prompt treatment of opportunistic infections. There remains no cure for HIV infection, but advances have been made both in preventing spread and in therapies used for this devastating disease.

Initially, health education programmes in the USA and Europe were aimed at changing the sexual behaviour of the homosexual communities. Their success seemed to be reflected by a drop in the incidence of other sexually transmitted diseases. Some infections such as gonorrhoea are now rising again in younger groups, so the impetus of these campaigns may now be less.

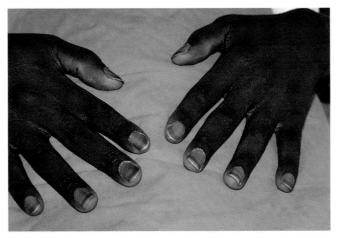

Fig. 140 Nail hyperpigmentation characteristic of long-term zidovudine therapy.

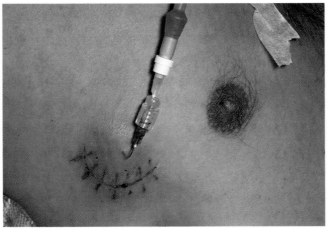

Fig. 141 Central line tunnelled into the subclavian vein for long-term intravenous drug therapy.

26 / **Prevention strategies**

Safer sex campaigns

Western countries have instituted campaigns via the media, government and voluntary agencies. HIV-antibody screening with pre- and post-test counselling is freely available in hospitals and the community. Education remains central to these programmes. The main message is: 'Reduce your number of sexual partners, know your partner's sexual and drug history, and use a condom'. In under-developed countries, however, there are major practical and cultural barriers to this approach (p. 107).

Needle-exchange units

Needle-exchange units provide sterile needles for intravenous drug users, and use the opportunity to educate. Where resources are limited or legislation limits needle exchange, household bleach has been distributed for needle cleaning.

Screening

Screening of donor blood, semen and organs has been employed in wealthier countries since 1985. These remain possible sources of HIV elsewhere.

Strategies against vertical transmission

These include barrier contraception, counselling 'at-risk' women of child-bearing age and avoidance of breast-feeding. Few of these are yet practical in Africa where communications are poor, and unsterile bottle-feeding is hazardous.

Protection of health care workers

Protection of health care workers also requires education. Phlebotomy (Fig. 142) should employ gloves and careful disposal of sharps. All spillages of body fluids should be cleaned with hypochlorite. Meticulous operating theatre protocol is essential (Fig. 143).

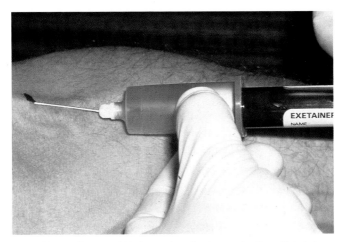

Fig. 142 The use of vacuum-phlebotomy reduces the chances of spillage of infected blood.

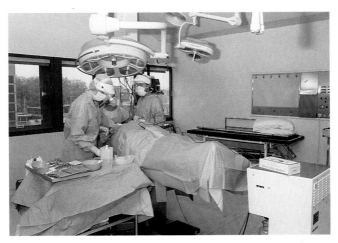

Fig. 143 Operating on a HIV-positive patient: double gloves, disposable gowns, drapes and masks.

Index